**Sascha Roos** is an author and dyslexia specialist in Cork, in the Republic of Ireland. She has been supporting people with the challenges of dyslexia for over fifteen years, and has an approach that encourages and cᴇ ebrates the strengths and abilities of the dyslexic individual.

Sasch s a member of the Dyslexia Association of Ireland and the Instit e of Guidance Counsellors. She has had articles published by natio dyslexia associations, including those of Britain, Australia and Irelaɪ and has a blog on study skills for dyslexic students for a leadiɪ study skills website. Her particular interest in the concerns and fɪ strations of parents and children with dyslexia drew her to write this g ide.

Sasch ontinues to work to transform the negative attitudes towards dyslex to raise expectations and to change the language around this learniɪ difference.

## Other titles

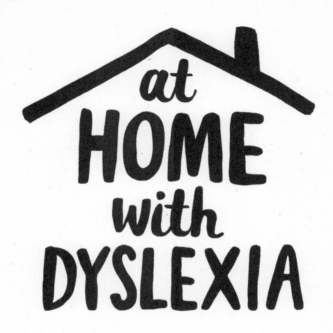

# at HOME with DYSLEXIA

## A Parent's Guide to Supporting Your Child

### SASCHA ROOS

Illustrations by Danielle Sheehy

ROBINSON

ROBINSON

First published in Great Britain in 2018 by
Robinson

Copyright © Sascha Roos, 2018
Illustrations copyright © Danielle Sheehy, 2018

3 5 7 9 10 8 6 4 2

IMPORTANT NOTE
The recommendations in this book are solely
intended as education and information and
should not be taken as medical advice.

A CIP catalogue record for this book
is available from the British Library.

ISBN: 978-1-47214-065-4

Typeset in Sentinel by
Initial Typesetting Services, Edinburgh
Printed and bound in Great Britain by
Clays Ltd, Elcograf S.p.A

Papers used by Robinson are from
well-managed forests and other responsible
sources

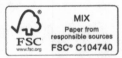

MIX
Paper from
responsible sources
FSC
www.fsc.org    FSC® C104740

Robinson
An imprint of
Little, Brown Book Group
Carmelite House
50 Victoria Embankment
London EC4Y 0DZ

An Hachette UK Company
www.hachette.co.uk

www.littlebrown.co.uk

For my uncle Bertie

'With dyslexia comes a very great gift, which is the way that your mind can think creatively. If your kids can be given the opportunity to find that way of thinking, what works for them, they will be very happy and successful in whatever field they choose to go into.'[1]

Orlando Bloom

# CONTENTS

# PREFACE

<u>At Home with Dyslexia: A Parent's Guide to Supporting your Child</u> is an up-to-date guide for parents wanting to know how they can best support their dyslexic child at home. It explores the areas of most concern to parents, with useful, day-to-day advice for practical and emotional support from the primary to secondary school years, as well as how to deal with the school and the education system.

There is a sea change in attitudes towards dyslexia, as shown in the growing numbers of famous and successful dyslexics speaking out about their own dyslexia. Successful dyslexics in all areas are communicating that, if addressed properly, dyslexia is not a problem; it can be recognized as an advantage. This is what parents want to hear.

In this guide, genuine encouragement of dyslexic abilities and strengths is supported by the success stories of dyslexic individuals in their own words. The personal accounts of dyslexic children and parents are woven throughout the chapters, where they share their experiences and advice in a reassuring and informative manner.

Dyslexia is regarded as genetic in origin, therefore this guide takes into consideration the likelihood that at least one parent will also be dyslexic. The structure and visual presentation of the book maintains the need to appeal to the dyslexic parent of the dyslexic child. Its 'dyslexia-friendly' appearance includes short chapters and paragraphs, bullet points, summaries and illustrations, making it an easy-to-follow guide that can be dipped into for useful tools and advice to help at home.

All references to 'parents' in the book naturally include other family members and carers of children with dyslexia.

Both boys and girls may be dyslexic, and this is reflected in the referencing of both boys' and girls' experiences throughout the book, giving a balance between genders.

As a powerful introduction to the changing attitudes towards dyslexia, Nicola, an art critic in New York, reflects with heartfelt honesty on her own experiences of having this learning difference. She shares her feelings about its challenges but also its rewards, and finally her hopes for the future that being dyslexic will be something to celebrate:

'For me, the term dyslexia has changed since I finished college and secondary school. At the beginning, I didn't know what to think, other than that it was a definition to do with the fact that I couldn't spell great or read to the level that I should. Yet I hated having the word stuck to me. When I was diagnosed with having dyslexia, people thought I had a disability, as the term "dyslexia" was still a "new thing" and people didn't know what to make of it. However, I have learned to know that it's not a disability as I am physically not disabled, yet it is still seen as a disability, which is infuriating.

'It doesn't affect our intelligence, which the majority of people don't understand. The main thing with dyslexia is that it is unique to everyone. Everyone's dyslexia affects each person differently, which in a way builds a little community, almost like a safe spot as we all "get it". We all understand how we feel. We are all comfortable around each other where there is no faking it or pretending that you don't have it.

'Dyslexia is challenging yet so rewarding! You have your days where you feel like you can master the world but, then, there are days where you can have such lows that you feel like everything you do is worthless. Dyslexia can be my best friend yet my biggest enemy.

'Overall, the last few years I have grown to love being dyslexic, yet I don't like to tell people that I have it unless I have to. In my opinion, even in the twenty-first century, there still is a taboo around dyslexia. Companies, schools and people don't know enough about it. They get embarrassed and shy away from it.

'I hope that dyslexia stops being referred to as a disability. It's not a disability but rather a learning difference which is unique to each and every one of us.'

'I think we need more famous actors, business people, chefs and other well-known people who have dyslexia to speak up about it and open the conversation about the challenges, as well as the great things that come with being dyslexic. This may result in other people feeling a bit more confident in having dyslexia and, thus, it may start to be seen in a different light.'

Nicola, art critic

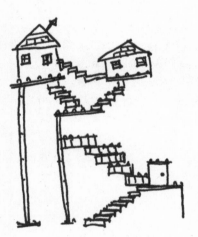

I couldn't
read the instructions,
So I made this!

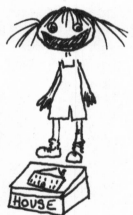

## CHAPTER ONE

# Understanding Dyslexia

'One very important thing to note from my point of view is that it is by no means a disability. I have always said that, because of my dyslexia, I think differently to others.'

Luke, engineer

This chapter provides an explanation of dyslexia, and how we can view dyslexia today. It looks at defining dyslexia by providing:

- a brief scientific analysis
- a rejection of the myths
- perspectives from dyslexics in their own words

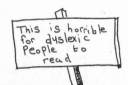

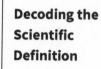

| The Scientific Bit: a Specific Learning Difficulty | Decoding the Scientific Definition |
|---|---|
| • 'Dyslexia is manifested in a continuum of specific learning difficulties related to the acquisition of basics skills in reading, spelling and/or writing; | • difficulties with learning reading, writing and spelling skills |
| • 'such difficulties being unexpected in relation to an individual's other abilities and educational experiences; | • difficulties not consistent with overall intelligence |
| • 'dyslexia can be described at the neurological, cognitive and behavioural levels. It is typically characterized by inefficient information processing, including difficulties in phonological processing, working memory, rapid naming and automaticity of basic skills; | • difficulties taking in information and with the sounds of letters, and matching sounds to words |
| • 'difficulties in organization and sequencing'.[1] | • difficulties remembering things in the short-term memory and learning by rote or off by heart |

## What is Dyslexia?

| Dyslexia <u>Is</u>: | Dyslexia Is <u>Not</u>: |
| --- | --- |
| • a learning difference | • a learning 'disability' |
| • an advantage | • an 'abnormality' |
| • occurring in people with average or above average IQ | • a product of low IQ; dyslexics are not stupid or slow |
| • an information-processing difference | • just a problem with reading and spelling |
| • a life-long 'condition' | • something one grows out of |
| • occurring in at least 8 per cent of the population from a mild to a severe degree | • the same for everyone; not all dyslexics are the same |

The best people to ask about dyslexia are those who have dyslexia. Here are some explanations from young people with dyslexia and their parents:

'It is just a different way of learning. I wouldn't say it is a disability; it's just a different way of looking at problem-solving. It's a myth that we can't read or write, that we're basically dumb. It's not a disability, we're not mentally impaired.'

Mike, graduate

'It's a difference from other people, not "special". We hate being called "special needs"!'

Sean, 13

'Just because I can't read, spell, learn and write as well as others doesn't mean that I'm not creatively minded.'

Claire, 14

'It is learning a different way . . . the ability to think differently. It is overcoming obstacles. It is knowing what hard work is.'

Emma, 17

'It is very individual, not one size fits all. It has nothing to do with intelligence.'

Maria, parent

'It is an inability to express on paper what they know in their head, understanding but not able to articulate the answer. Dyslexics are powerfully intuitive, very intelligent, have an amazing ability to hide the problems that dyslexia causes, but on the other hand the short-term memory is very iffy.'

Elmarie, parent

'It should be seen as a positive difference. It is another way of thinking and learning.'

Françoise, parent

**'I think dyslexia is an extraordinary characteristic, and it is certainly not something that needs to be fixed, or cured, or suppressed! We think outside the box precisely because we have never been in one.'[2]**

**Jack Horner, palaeontologist**

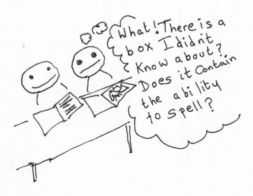

The word **'dyslexia'** is derived from the Greek language:

**dys** = difficult

**lexis** = word

**lexia** = reading

**Dys-lex-ia** - the word itself is very limiting. It's a term that doesn't truly encompass the experiences of a dyslexic individual. We know that dyslexia is a difficulty with reading, spelling and writing and other aspects of language, but what else is it?

## Dyslexia is a different wiring of the brain

**CASE STUDY**

**TADHG, 15**

'We're not slow, we're different. You think in different ways – better ways than other people even.

'You need a different way of thinking, if everyone thought with the left side of the brain then everything would be like half the world – it would be straight on. Without the dyslexics it wouldn't be so creative, it would be a different world. I think it's an advantage really, only 8 per cent of people think the way you do, and then there's the 92 per cent that think the other way, and you may feel that your opinion is not valued, but actually without it the world wouldn't function – Leonardo da Vinci, all that he created, Edison, Darwin, Gates, Ford – there would be no evolution, light bulbs, telephone, all the biggest inventions, things you see everywhere – there would be no electricity, cars, laptops . . . we couldn't stay in contact with everyone in the world.'

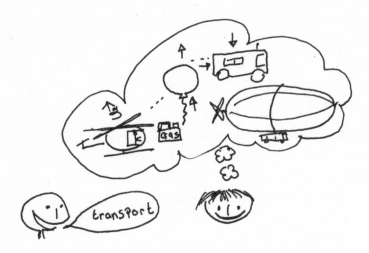

## The Dyslexic Brain Is Different

There is enough scientific evidence now to show that the dyslexic brain processes information differently. Through brain-scanning techniques, neuroscience can show how the dyslexic brain is more active in the right hemisphere, and has some connection differences with the left hemisphere. So the challenges for someone with dyslexia are largely due to these differences in the left hemisphere and the areas of the brain that deal with language skills – the process of enabling reading and writing does not work as efficiently as for the non-dyslexic brain.

However, the discovery of the more symmetrical right and left hemispheres of the dyslexic brain gives an added advantage for the dyslexic. This symmetry and different activity of the dyslexic brain is good news for the dyslexic individual, and explains the abilities that stand out compared to struggles in other areas for the dyslexic child.

## Dyslexia Is a Different Ability

The most important aspect of dyslexia for you to remember is that it is a pattern of weaknesses and strengths, a processing difference. It is a different pattern of brain organization and information processing which will predispose a dyslexic individual to the development of certain valuable skills.

Dyslexia should be seen as a different learning ability rather than a disability. Dyslexia is not something you 'have' or 'suffer with'; it is part of who you are. It is a way of thinking, learning and seeing the world.

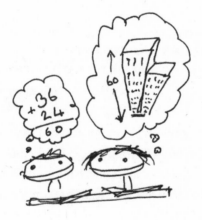

'It's good fun having a brain that can keep yourself entertained. It means you can do a whole load of things other people can't do.'

Danielle, parent with dyslexia

'It's having difficulty with academic aspects but it's not remotely affecting your intelligence, so you can still comprehend and be perfectly intelligent but have dyslexia at the same time. In other aspects it is a bit of a gift. It has allowed me to be more driven. I do think that dyslexia has given me skills that have benefited me in every aspect. It's a different way of seeing things. It's not a disability, it's not an illness, it is not a diagnosis.'

Katie, graduate with dyslexia

The dyslexic brain has its own kind of strengths, benefits and advantages which should be recognized and enjoyed. Our goal is to help a dyslexic individual recognize these advantages and enjoy the full range of benefits that can come from the dyslexic brain.

> 'It's not a disability, it's an attribute . . . I feel I can do anything, it helps me.'
>
> Luke, engineer

> **'Us dyslexic people, we've got it going on — we are the architects. We are the designers. I always say, "Bloody non-dyslexics . . . who do they think they are?"'[3]**
>
> **Benjamin Zephaniah, poet**

Yes, this guide book is mainly to support parents with the challenges and difficulties a dyslexic child faces through his school career, but we must also emphasize his dyslexic talents. We must think more broadly about what it really means to be dyslexic and that it no longer means only challenges but also includes important talents and strengths.

Knowing that the skills and capacities of the dyslexic child are as significant in our view of dyslexia as its challenges is something to keep in mind throughout your use of this book.

## Takeaways from Chapter 1

- know what dyslexia really is
- see the difficulties but also the strengths

## CHAPTER TWO

# How Do I Know If My Child Has Dyslexia?

'Often best mates are dyslexic – they find each other – they're like me, I'm like him, we're all like my dad. It's a feeling . . . we'll have a conversation that others wouldn't grasp but would make total sense to us.'

Tadhg, 15

This chapter will look at how to spot dyslexia from early childhood to the teenage years. It focuses on the inherent difficulties as well as strengths by presenting:

- possible signs in language development, reading and writing skills
- symptoms of short-term memory and sequencing difficulties
- common feelings and character traits
- typical strengths and abilities

## Trusting Your Intuition

Parents are best placed to be on the alert for early signs of dyslexia. But before we look at signs in the early years, here are three points to note:

<u>Trust the feelings</u> you may be having that there is something 'different' about your child but you can't quite explain what it is.

'Go with your gut instinct.'

Ann, parent

'I would get annoyed at the lack of progress I was making. My advice is pay attention to your child's progress. If you notice there are certain things they excel at and certain things that are not quite as advanced as they should be, like forgetting certain sentences or how things are structured or the sound of things, trust your "gut feeling".'

Mike, graduate

<u>Look at genetic evidence</u> – there is much well-documented research to show that dyslexia is hereditary. So look at family history – not just parents and siblings, but also grandparents, uncles, aunts and cousins.

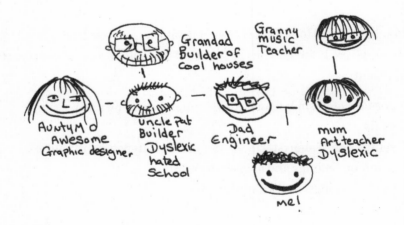

'She's like me! I wasn't aware what to look out for. When you're living with it, it's hard to spot. Go with your gut feeling.'

Danielle, dyslexic parent

However, when thinking about spotting the signs of dyslexia, be aware that an individual child won't have all the symptoms, and two dyslexics in the same family may have very different experiences.

<u>Don't worry or feel bad if you are coming to dyslexia later in your child's development</u> – although it is true that early spotting and intervention is invaluable for the dyslexic child, you are here now and that's the main thing. Be aware it is certainly possible for the difficulties of a very bright child or a quiet child to go unnoticed as long as their progress is more or less average.

> 'Reading, writing and especially spelling were the most challenging aspects of learning in school for me. The most prevalent feeling for me was one of frustration. My reading and writing age was continually two years behind my actual age, while I scored in some of the highest percentiles in spatial, problem-solving and mathematics. At an early age, it was frustrating not to be recognized for my actual intelligence and ability in school.'
>
> Luke, engineer

## Spotting the Signs – the Early Years (ages 3-7)

### Language development

Language development is a challenge for many young children with dyslexia and a significant feature in its identification.

- Phonological processing and awareness is the greatest challenge, which means being able to recognize individual sounds in words and to distinguish between word sounds. For example: vowel sound difference between 'i' and 'e' as in 'pit' and 'pet'; and 'u' and 'o' as in 'cut' and 'cot'
- Language delay (however, not always; they can be articulate with good verbal skills from an early age)

- Word naming problems and inventing words for things
- Spoonerisms – jumbling words. For example: 'parcark', 'flutterby'
- Struggling with learning nursery rhymes
- Difficulty retrieving words to express themselves
- Slow to master the use of tenses
- Mispronouncing longer words

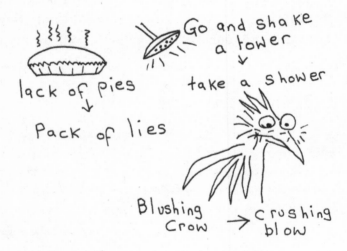

'I remember learning "ch" and "sh" sounds – it didn't make sense, but other kids had it and already knew it. Why do these letters make that noise? It doesn't make sense!'

Leah, 19, remembering her early primary school years

**Sequencing and working memory (short-term memory)**
Challenges may include:

- learning to dress
- learning nursery rhymes
- following routines
- following a set of instructions
- repeating messages

- remembering what they did in school today
- remembering spellings for tests
- learning times tables
- learning the alphabet, days of the week, months of the year

'Our daughter did very well up until 1st class [around six or seven years old], where actual rote learning is beginning. She struggled with spellings, so my advice is watch out for the ability to spell correctly on the day, but everything completely forgotten about by the next day or even hour. Same goes with tables. The Drumcondra test [a standardized test] was an eye opener as she clearly did very badly in it.'

Elmarie, parent

'I'd have to say the alphabet in my head, sing the whole tune of it to know where the letter was, and other people would just know it.'

Leah, 19, remembering her early primary school years

'Everywhere we'd go in the car, my dad would always ask me the tables, but in two days I'd just forget them. I don't know them now! The clock took years to learn. I still don't know the 24-hour clock.'

Juliette, 17, remembering her early primary school years

## The skill of reading

The skill of reading can be a huge challenge and an almost insurmountable task, which can affect the dyslexic throughout her life. Early recognition and intervention will make an enormous difference, and may open doors and a love of reading that a dyslexic child would not have found without that intervention.

Look out for these signs in a dyslexic child's first attempts to read:

- Problems with phonological processing, which means struggling to recognize letter symbols and their sounds

- Difficulty reading single words in isolation without context clues
- Poor word attack skills, especially for new words
- Confusing small words and reversing words, for example: 'how'/'who'; 'form'/'from'; 'was'/'saw'
- Enjoying being read to but showing no desire to pick up a book and learn to read
- Relying on pictures and contextual clues
- Using clever tactics to appear to be reading. For example: memorizing the text from hearing it previously
- Getting the initial letter and guessing the rest of the word
- Reading aloud is slow, choppy and laborious
- Omitting words, adding words, substituting a word for a similar-looking word or meaning. For example: 'collapse'/'capsize'

'I didn't understand why it took me longer to learn than others. It was clear I found reading challenging at a young age. My advice is parents should look out for signs of their children getting frustrated, if their child hates school because they find it hard, if they constantly can't keep up with class mates.'

Emma, 17, remembering her primary school years

'I remember getting upset because I couldn't concentrate on what I was reading and my mum was telling me to hurry up. I didn't know why the others weren't struggling as much as I was. That's when my mum and dad tried to figure out what it was. Try to understand and figure out what's wrong with your child. My mum didn't have a clue and when she found out it was much easier and we could figure out what to do.'

Aoife, 13, remembering her early primary school years

'I definitely couldn't read! I was so frustrated. I'd be reading each word individually but not engaging the meaning to the brain. I avoided reading a lot.'

Molly, 19, remembering her early primary school years

## Parents' advice from their experiences of the early primary school years

'Look for problems with reading and phonetics, look for distress and unease in school or with school work. Watch to see if your child has understanding verbally but goes blank when attempting reading tasks.'

Lisa, parent of two dyslexic daughters

'It just wasn't the focus in early infants to learn and match the sounds to the letters. This became more apparent as a "problem" around 2nd and 3rd class [between seven and nine years old] when reading was slow, spelling was not retained and my daughter could not write independently, mixing up the letters even in the simplest and smallest words.'

Liz

'He just didn't pick up phonics in junior infants. In hindsight, all those interventions in school and yet dyslexia was still not on the radar. If your child is getting extra help in school then pursue the dyslexia avenue.'

Yvonne, parent of three dyslexic sons

## Spotting the Signs – the Later Primary School Years (ages 8–11)

### Reading

Reading difficulties become more acute as time goes on for the dyslexic child:

- Reading achievement is below expectations, approximately two years below the expected level for age and ability
- Reluctance to read aloud
- Ignoring the significance of full stops and commas when reading aloud

- Skipping lines and words, and losing place frequently
- Preferring to use a finger, pen or marker to help follow the words
- Relying on sight vocabulary (words that are learnt and instantly recognized) rather than breaking down a new word to its individual sounds
- Clever tactics to avoid reading
- Finding reading a greater effort and more tiring than their siblings
- Having to read a passage several times to comprehend its meaning

'We'd have loads of books around the house. I didn't want to read the book but I wanted to know the story. I'd take away the book and try to read it myself. I didn't want to read it in front of Mum or Dad because it was embarrassing, I couldn't properly read it.'

Katie, 19, remembering her primary school years

'I used strategies to avoid reading – I'd get my sister to read for me. I'd spend ages, double the amount of time another child would.'

Leah, 19, remembering her primary school years

'I used to lie about how many books I read. I hated reading. I absolutely despised it. I only read one book.'

Jennifer, 18, remembering her primary school years

'If they're not interested in it at all, see what that's about.'

14-year-old Caoimhe's sage advice about reading

## Irlen Syndrome or Scotopic Sensitivity

If your child complains of glare from a white page, the words moving or blurring and has frequent headaches from reading, then consider looking into this visual perception difficulty. It is sensitivity to specific frequencies in the light spectrum, undetected by a conventional eye test. Some people with dyslexia are also known to have this perception difficulty alongside their dyslexia, or they may be misdiagnosed as dyslexic, their Irlen Syndrome or Scotopic Sensitivity remaining undetected.

> 'I felt as if it took me longer and I lost concentration a lot. The spaces were big between words. Everyone thinks that dyslexia is words moving on the page, but this is not the case. My coloured lenses really helped. I used to suffer from headaches when I read but the lenses have completely cured that and also make it easier to read.'
>
> Emma, 17

Trust your gut feeling, talk to your child and look into Irlen Syndrome if you feel it may be part of the jigsaw. (See more on this visual perception difficulty in the Appendix).

## Spelling

Things to look out for:

- Doing reasonably well in spelling tests but only after a lot of preparation and drilling
- The same spellings won't be recalled two days later
- Still making basic mistakes with everyday words. For example, strong indicators include: 'how'/'who'; 'dose'/'does'; 'wich'/'which'; 'feel'/'fell'
- Confusing vowel sounds. For example: 'mat'/'met'; 'cut'/'cot'
- Breaking down words to syllables can be a challenge, adding too many syllables to a word, or too few. For example: 'sundly' instead of 'suddenly'
- Spelling a word differently on the same page and not noticing
- Not being able to spot their own spelling errors
- Reversing letters beyond the age you would expect, particularly 'b'/'d' confusion

- Even though they appear highly articulate and able to grasp concepts quickly, they cannot comprehend unorthodox spellings such as silent letters – because for them there is no logic in these spellings

---

**CASE STUDY**

**KATIE, 19, REMEMBERING HER STRUGGLES WITH SPELLING**

'I can definitely remember . . . why wasn't I getting remotely near the person who was sitting to the left of me or to the right? And asking my mum, "Is there something wrong with me?"

'I used to get awfully confused with my b's and d's, so I did that "bed" thing and that used to be written at the top of all my books to remind myself. And my teacher would ask my mum, "Why is bed written on everything?" They didn't realize at all.'

---

'Her letter-forming seems to have a lot of reversals.'

Cathal, parent

'Spellings she would learn every day for her weekly spelling test would be forgotten by Friday morning, so basically she gave up.'

Colleen, parent

## Writing

A clear indicator of dyslexia can be found in examples of free writing by a dyslexic child – those pieces of creative writing about their holidays or their pet. Why, after great discussion on the subject, have they only written three lines? You know they have potential but it just isn't being translated to their written work.

Signs to look out for, particularly in their free writing:

- Can describe a story orally very competently, yet enormous difficulty transferring this story on to the page
- Avoidance, frustration and tears until a very simple paragraph is produced, which the teacher puts down to laziness
- Confusing tenses between past and present in free writing
- Confusing third person and first person in a story (from 'he' to 'I')
- Difficulty with grammar rules and word order
- Can never remember nouns, adjectives or verbs
- Still finding capital letters and full stops hard to master, and commas are a mystery
- Using a restricted vocabulary of words they believe they can spell

'I remember not being able to do things, not a clue what to do! So my friend would let me copy hers.'

Molly, 19, remembering writing at primary school

'I couldn't write the sentence in the time given, I just wouldn't get to the answer.'

Sarah, 15, remembering her primary school years

'I find it hard to get the story just written on to the page. Sometimes I'd have it in my mind but actually writing it is very hard.'

Luca, 10

## Teacher observations in the primary classroom – what to look out for

Some points that teachers may bring up with you, but without possibly making the link to dyslexia:

- Difficulty learning the names and sounds of letters and breaking down words to their sounds. For example: 'sh-o-p'
- Needing a lot of repetition of a word before it becomes known and used accurately and consistently
- Needing time to process information and respond
- Labelled as having poor concentration, easily distracted and doesn't seem to listen in class
- Relying on a limited sight vocabulary and not making the transition to decoding unfamiliar but quite basic words
- Reading comprehension is below what is expected for their intelligence, as evident in class discussion
- Misinterpreting questions in their school tests
- Written work lacking structure, not enough care over spellings (red pen all over the page)
- Not retaining the times tables
- Progress is inconsistent

'I wasn't good at listening. It was the same at every parent–teacher meeting. I couldn't believe it when they said that I was lacking listening skills, even though I was trying so hard, but it was in one ear and out the other. I really wanted to be interested but it wouldn't go in and stay in.'

Abbie, 14, remembering her primary school years

'My advice is to ask at parent–teacher meetings, "Where does that put her in her age group?" I was struggling but I was still participating in class and able to comprehend what was going on. I was really interactive with hands-on things. I was really willing to learn and the teacher recognized that.'

Katie, remembering her primary school experiences

'I always got the same comments on my reports: 'Try harder' . . . 'Not working to her best ability'.

Caoimhe, 14, remembering her primary school years

'My son was diagnosed in 5th class [around ten years old] in primary school. He had consistently low grades in his annual STen tests ['standard ten' tests that gather information on the level of your child's reading and maths ability] but the teachers thought that he wasn't concentrating properly.'

Mary, parent

'If I missed something everyone else was learning, it would take me a long time to get to where everyone else was. I didn't know the steps.'

Helena, 12, remembering her primary school experience

## Secondary School and the Teenage Years

**CASE STUDY**

**NIAMH'S EXPERIENCES WITH HER DYSLEXIC DAUGHTER**

'What would I advise other parents to look out for? I would say look out for the obvious spelling mistakes, even though your child may have spelt everything correctly one day, yet inexplicably getting it wrong the next. Or getting very basic, simple words wrong, and not realizing they are wrong at all until it is pointed out, and weirdly, in our case, not caring that they are spelt wrong!

'I would say look out for a certain sense of lack of organization, as in when they are trying to think ahead in terms of organization, or following a time-frame for something, seeming to be not "clued in" to the amount or lack of time in which to do something.

'I would also look out for a marked change in being a perfectly capable student in primary to becoming "distracted", "scatty" in secondary, as was said about my daughter. It was the whole new concept of following a timetable, different rooms, different teachers for different subjects, having to be organized for the next and the next class, not quite "getting it", long after most other students would have eventually settled into secondary school, seeming to be still overwhelmed by everything that is so new and different.

'I would also look out for not being too keen on reading books, or anything wordy, even posters or signs, or articles online, or out and about, as in our case, at the Titanic Exhibition in Cobh, which was where the first penny dropped for me . . .'

It is quite possible for dyslexia to go unnoticed throughout primary and even up to the senior cycle in secondary school. Do not despair if you are coming to dyslexia at this late stage. As mentioned at the beginning of the chapter, the signs of dyslexia may be masked by the hard work and concentration of the child, and might only become evident when the challenges and pressures of secondary school bring these underlying difficulties to the fore.

## Possible Indicators at Secondary School

### Difficulties with reading and writing

- unable to skim or scan for information, they have to read the whole piece again to find the relevant information
- still lacking fluency in reading
- proofreading is impossible – they just can't see their own errors
- still can't get the hang of paragraphs
- commas remain a mystery
- avoid attempting more challenging words for fear of the difficult spelling, therefore their actual intelligence is not reflected in their written expression
- can't plan or structure essays

- answers to questions are slightly off the mark
- sentence structure can be awkward, not using connecting words efficiently
- their written work never reflects their verbal intelligence
- continue to experience spelling difficulties
- their class notes aren't clear, they can't get everything down in time in class
- often don't get the homework written down correctly
- can't quite pull the word they want out of their head
- need a bit more time to process their thoughts on the information they are receiving
- labelled 'lazy', 'careless', 'not concentrating'
- despite putting in tremendous effort, they have little to show for it

'I knew there was something wrong but didn't know what it was. I knew there was something different but not in a good way. I'd put so much into exams and never get results.'

Jennifer, 18, found out she was dyslexic at 15

'I could always speak a story but could never write them. I'd have an essay in my head but only get ten lines on the page and that was always really frustrating. I would never get it from my head to the page. Teachers would say, "That's not good enough, do it again."'

Tadhg, 15

'The key sign I found that made me think that she could be dyslexic was the difficulty she had taking down homework from the board in school.'

Colleen, parent

## The issues with memory
Poor memory is the biggest frustration at secondary school and a sure sign of dyslexia. Specific signs might be:

- Persistently being punished for forgetting books and homework, even though they are desperately using tactics to try to remember
- Struggling with conventional learning techniques
- Poor memory for recent events, like the exam yesterday
- Can't learn sequences by rote (off by heart), like in Science
- Impossible to learn quotes in English studies
- Need to read a passage several times to digest the contents
- Can't retain the new vocabulary of subjects
- Learning languages is a huge challenge, particularly spelling and grammar
- Having a working memory overload, resulting in frustration and stress

'My short-term memory affects me a lot.'

Sean, 13

'It's the detail I can't remember.'

Owen, 18

**CASE STUDY**

**JULIETTE, 17, REFLECTING ON HER POOR SHORT-TERM MEMORY**

'I was always making the same mistakes, never bringing the right books, and the teacher sending notes home and punishing me for being scattered. I'd do my homework and forget my copybook at home, I was so annoyed.

'My mum had to come in all the time with my lunchbox. And when the school needed a parent's signature, I would think, "Oh yeah, I must get that signed," but as soon as I got home I'd never remember it again. My mum would say, "You didn't give me the note . . . how am I supposed to know about the school tour!"'

'Spot when your child is forgetting stuff, bringing the wrong books home, reading the timetable wrongly. If I didn't write things down in my homework journal it would be forgotten in an hour. I'd get a note home saying I hadn't done my homework but I'd forgotten to write it down.'

Katie, 19

## Spotting the Signs at Any Age

At all ages, a major sign is the sheer exhaustion dyslexic children feel at the end of a school day, compared to their siblings and peers. On Fridays, they collapse with exhaustion after a week of school; in half-term breaks, they just want to sleep. Students with dyslexia have to work four times harder than other students to keep on top of the reading, note-taking, learning and so on. Some recognizable signs are:

- being exhausted after a long day in school
- being easily distracted
- capable of being focused when driven to be
- having random thoughts
- being unaware of time
- not being able to see the wood for the trees
- symptoms increasing with stress, time pressure and tiredness
- having good days and bad days
- struggling with poor self-esteem

'I was really tired in school and would be nearly falling asleep in class.'

Caoimhe, 14

'He is very easily distracted and finds it difficult to concentrate. He becomes frustrated very easily.'

Mary, parent

'Before I was diagnosed, I felt useless, I felt stupid and I could feel people judge me when I would read aloud. It was challenging when

I couldn't get the words to come out of my mouth and it made me feel like a tiny curled-up ball. I would advise parents to look out for low self-esteem in their child and I would watch out for frustration in spelling and reading.'

Claire, 14

'I thought I was slow, my parents didn't know I felt like that. I thought it was a normal feeling. I didn't tell anybody. They didn't think anything was wrong with me because I was very good at other things. I was good at Maths and Sport, and Maths judges people's intelligence more than English.'

Tadhg, 15

'Look out for your child saying, "I'm the worst in the class," when she comes home from school.'

Danielle's advice as a parent

Ask your child how they're feeling. And then <u>listen</u>.

'I always thought there was something.'

Alex discovered she had dyslexia aged 17

'Listen to your child if they feel they need to be tested. A friend asked her mum to get her tested and she said, "No, you're fine."'

Caoimhe, 14

## Recognizing Strengths

'The connection between dyslexia and creativity makes me go off in strange directions and make sideways connections.'[1]

Eddie Izzard, comedian, actor, writer

As you have seen in Chapter 1, dyslexia is a different way of seeing the world, a different wiring of the brain, a right-hemisphere emphasis.

There will, therefore, be a pattern of strengths and weaknesses for the dyslexic individual, certain talents that may well stand out compared to difficulties with relatively simple tasks.

Alongside the struggles you are spotting in your dyslexic child, do not overlook certain skills and talents, those stand-out abilities which may also be a sign of dyslexia – the creative, inherent aspects of a child with dyslexia.

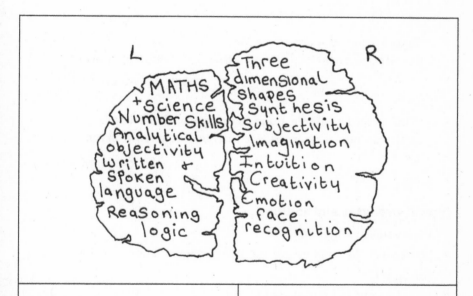

| **Left-brained** | **Right-brained** |
| --- | --- |
| verbal | visual-spatial |
| language oriented | experience oriented |
| analytical | holistic, creative |
| sequential | random |
| linear | global |
| logical | free flowing |
| rational | intuitive |
| time oriented | timeless |

'The dyslexic brain has two sides; one is smart and the other is all over the place!'

Sean, 13

Here are the views of possibly two of the most famous individuals in history with dyslexia. Albert Einstein and Leonardo da Vinci recognized their abilities and made sure their talents propelled them forward, so much so that we continue to be affected by their different ways of seeing the world to this day.

'Imagination is more important than knowledge. Knowledge is limited. Imagination encircles the world.'

Albert Einstein

'You should prefer a good scientist without literary abilities than a literate one without scientific skills.'

Leonardo da Vinci

## Typical strengths and abilities

- verbal intelligence, articulate
- creative ideas, vivid imagination (although not easily transferred to the page)
- gifted at maths, mental arithmetic, mathematical concepts
- superior reasoning
- visual-spatial strength
- ability to recognize patterns
- talented in art and making things
- talented in drama, storytelling
- talented in music, dance
- talented in sport, team playing
- talented in mechanics, fixing things

- good problem-solving, grasping the bigger picture
- divergent thinking, originality
- excellent long-term memory for certain things

'Look at what they are really good at – the difference between two subjects, different skills. Being a good liar! On the spot they can think of excuses, verbally good but not at writing down stuff. I have an opinion on everything!'

Tadhg, 15

'I'm good at Maths, it's structured and ordered. Maths was one of my strengths and I really succeeded in Maths. English has no order, it's crazy.'

Mike, graduate

'I have always said my abilities are because of my dyslexia. I was classed as a "gifted" child and had a high aptitude for problem-solving, mathematics and excellent spatial awareness. Again, I accredit my intelligence to being dyslexic and thinking differently because of this.'

Luke, engineer

'Thanks to my dyslexia I'm good at seeing patterns in things.'

Sean, 13

'I do much more intricate designs in Art compared to others. I have a great eye for colour.'

Aoibhinn, 14

'I loved sport and being involved. I was team captain at school and I was good at motivating people. I was really on the ball in being a team leader, organizing and delegating. I'm a team player; I see solutions and ways round.'

Katie, 19

## Some common characteristics

- observant, curious
- a busy mind
- intuitive, perceptive
- endurance and commitment to a task (when interested)
- empathy
- strong interpersonal skills
- not following the crowd

> 'She is very creative, observant and measured in her observations. Quietly absorbs a lot of detail of her surroundings.'
>
> Liz, parent

> 'I think I am more creative than other people, I like singing and music. I'm friendly, I'm more compassionate to people because if someone is struggling I can understand how they feel, I can empathize and help them.'
>
> Alex, 18

> 'My mum says I'm good at figuring out stuff.'
>
> Anna, 9

## Takeaways from Chapter 2

- trust your gut feeling
- look for signs in reading and writing
- ask your child
- don't forget to spot the strengths

## CHAPTER THREE

# I Think My Child Has Dyslexia ... What Next?

'Follow your instinct.'

Françoise, parent

This chapter will explore the option of a formal assessment for dyslexia and how to make the most of the results by:

- arranging an assessment as soon as possible
- preparing for the appointment
- understanding the report
- using the report effectively to support your child

So you have trusted your 'gut feeling', you have listened to class teachers and learning support teachers and you have listened to your child. And perhaps you can spot yourself in your child.

You are pretty sure that your child has dyslexia. What next? This is crunch time for a parent – what is the best course of action for your child, for you, for your family? Above all, it's important that you:

- don't panic
- don't overreact

- don't ignore
- don't delay

Don't delay in exploring the range of support open to your child, hopefully formalized, with the recommendations included in a professional educational psychologist's report.

## The Importance of a Professional Assessment

Parents who have been through this process give their advice on getting a professional assessment as soon as possible:

'Parents should take advice from teachers and not take offence if they are concerned about your child. So many parents ignore very important advice. An assessment is vital.'

Therese

'If possible, get on to the school's schedule for a psychological assessment. Tell them you want an assessment; do not wait for it to be offered. If they can't do it, do it anyway, pay for it, get it done. I hated the idea of a label but it was this assessment that allows you to get things done. The sooner you have the assessment, the sooner you can start to get help.'

Cathal

'First port of call has to be an assessment. Try to get a recommendation from another parent.'

Lisa

## Key Players in Early Identification

- The parents – they are in the best position to spot the signs (see chapter 2)

- Health professionals, speech therapists
- Educational professionals – the pre-school carer, the class teacher, the learning support assistant

Pressure for recognition of a child's difficulties is parent-driven. With children from as young as three or four years old, parents can have a feeling that 'something isn't quite right', particularly if they recognize their own younger self's difficulties in their child. It is possible to identify areas
of weakness and difficulty in these pre-school years, and parents can ask for an informal assessment, or 'screening', from as young as four years old.

If you feel there is reason for concern, screening tests can be given by the class teacher or special needs teacher. They can help spot a child's learning strengths and weaknesses and implement an individual education plan.

All children develop at different rates, so a reading delay may not mean dyslexia is the answer. It is important to communicate all concerns with the class teacher and ask for further investigation and screening by the school, before taking the next step towards an educational psychologist's assessment.

Many parents, particularly those with a family history of dyslexia, have a good idea when dyslexia is there. However, a full assessment for a 'specific learning difficulty' can't really be carried out until a child is seven or eight years old. It is then that you can pursue a definitive assessment for dyslexia. And, unfortunately, 'pursue' is often exactly the case in parents' experiences. They must pursue a psychologist's assessment through the school's system, or resort to an assessment from a professional working privately. Sadly, this is often the route parents must take if they want a prompt and detailed assessment with recommendations.

Schools are over-stretched and invariably lacking funds. The child with possible dyslexia who is just about coping in school will be way down the list for the visiting educational psychologist from the Department of Education. Individuals with behavioural problems will be prioritized, and parents could be waiting two years or more for that definitive report their child needs.

> 'An early-as-possible educational psychologist's report is essential so that you can fully understand your child's abilities and areas where extra help is required. School assessments are limited by funding so there can be significant financial implications to trying to get the best help and resources for your child.'
>
> Colleen's experience as a parent

### The importance of early intervention

If your dyslexic child is offered the correct support as young as possible, then there is less need for catching up and fewer feelings of frustration and failure. If the child's difficulties are not recognized and given the necessary support, then your child may fall behind more and more while others in the class surge ahead.

So much of the damage to self-confidence and self-image later on can be avoided, and emotional and behavioural problems prevented, if prompt and appropriate intervention is made in early childhood. Unfortunately, parents are reliant on the professionals' awareness and understanding of dyslexia. Sometimes, you just can't wait for your child's teacher to spot dyslexia, you have to identify it yourself and insist on the appropriate support.

Dyslexic students reflecting on early intervention:

> 'It would have helped if I'd known that I had dyslexia sooner, so at least then I'd know I wasn't slow.'
>
> Abbie

> 'I was much better equipped to deal with mistakes than my siblings diagnosed at a later age.'
>
> Niamh

> 'Once dyslexia is flagged, get the report done. No point leaving it 'til later in secondary school . . . by then the student will have so many coping mechanisms, whoever has to deal with them will have to deconstruct them and build them back up again.'
>
> Mike

## Why is a full professional report so important?

Parents relate their experiences of having a detailed report of their child's difficulties, strengths and recommended support strategies:

> 'I felt that the assessment and the diagnosis was a relief. There was a reason behind everything, and the homework became less stressful for everyone! It is the best money I have ever spent!'
>
> Ann

> 'Getting the assessment was very important for my son because it changed his whole experience of education. He received extra support in school and felt more comfortable with his teachers because he now felt there was a reason for his learning problems.'
>
> Mary

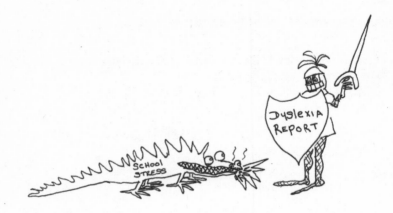

'It's a very good negotiating tool. The support of a psychologist gives you power.'

Dolores

## Preparing for an Educational Psychologist's Assessment

Don't be daunted by the idea of a 'psychologist'. This doesn't mean Freudian analysis. It means a professional who can administer tests that will find your child's IQ (intelligence quotient) and any discrepancies between abilities in some areas and weaknesses in others, which then do not correspond with your child's overall average or above-average IQ.

There are many dyslexics out there who are eligible to join MENSA (members must have an IQ of at least 130). So don't fear these tests; they will be far more accurate than any of the standardized tests that your child has to complete as part of the Department of Education's way of judging children's ability.

### A note about standardized tests

Standardized testing for children is part of the modern school experience, and often is carried out at specific points in a child's school career, for example at seven and eleven years old. It is important to know that these tests have limitations for children with dyslexia. It will be difficult to receive an accurate result for the dyslexic child who is bright, but needs more time to read and process a sequence of instructions in the time allowed.

<u>It is key to remember not to rely on standardized tests as a measure of a dyslexic child's ability or potential</u>. An educational psychologist's assessment is far more valid an instrument for assessing your child's ability. And don't allow teachers who work with your child to assume such tests confirm low ability.

Therefore, it is extremely important that a full professional report's findings are shared with the school and all teachers so that a dyslexic child's real potential can be recognized. The significance of a full psycho-educational report must not be underestimated when too often these standardized tests place children with dyslexia as low achievers destined for the weaker classes at secondary school.

## Being prepared for the assessment

---

**CASE STUDY**

**KATIE'S EXPERIENCE AT THE AGE OF 10**

'The first time when I went to the educational psychologist I felt so traumatized by it all. It was one of the scariest days of my life. I just didn't really understand what was going on. In my mind, I was being taken somewhere to be tested. It was very formal and straight away my mum and I were split up and I was very nervous. My experience of tests was always so horrible, I was getting all flustered. I was trying so hard.'

---

The assessment needn't be a scary experience for a child, and Katie's feelings could be avoided with some preparation:

- If you are pursuing an assessment outside school, aim to find an educational psychologist recommended by another parent.
- Find out as much as you can about the assessment procedure in advance.
- Make a note of any questions you want to ask.
- Be honest – explain to your child as best you can where you are going and why it will be a positive thing to do.
- Know its purpose – to identify strengths as well as difficulties, and provide direction for both parents and teachers on how best to support your child.
- Make sure your child doesn't think it is a test to confirm how stupid he feels but will, in fact, assess how he thinks and learns and show his true potential.
- Remember it is not an exam, there is no pass or fail.
- For older children, it can determine the type and level of support required for the state exams and beyond to university.

**What to expect during the assessment**

The assessment aims to gather as much information as possible on your child. Parents are asked questions about their child's early development, eyesight, hearing and so on. It is then best if parents leave the assessment tests so as not to distract or inhibit the process.

The psychologist will guide your child through tasks which will give overall ability, working memory, verbal and visual-spatial ability, as well as tests to assess levels of reading, comprehension, spelling, written expression and mathematics.

Your child or teenager may well become absorbed by the assessment and find it quite interesting and enjoyable, after the initial trepidation. The main thing is for you to convey a relaxed attitude and a confidence that this will be a step towards helping your child with her difficulties.

The psychologist will have a good idea whether there are any specific learning difficulties present, but will probably prefer to work on the report before giving any definitive results. Parents should expect to receive the full written report usually within a four- to six-week period.

## Understanding the Completed Assessment

A report is written with various readers in mind – teachers and other professionals, as well as the parents. Therefore, the language of the report can appear quite complex and daunting for the family. Parents should always feel that they can ask for feedback and clarification of any confusing parts of the report.

To add to this sometimes impenetrable professional jargon, a parent with dyslexia looks at these pages of dense black-and-white print and may find it difficult to pinpoint the key findings of the report – what is important to know, what actions they need to take.

There will be a variety of approaches professionals take to structure their reports, and some will be more formal and technical than others. Here are some probable sections of the report and its professional terms:

Background – reasons why an assessment was requested, family history of difficulties, teachers' reports, difficulties observed as well as strengths. The report is confidential but will be read by teachers and other professionals, so indicate if there are any details you would rather were not written into the report.

Tests administered – for example the Wechsler Intelligence Scale for

Children (WISC) gives an overall measure of a child's level of intellectual (cognitive) ability, the full-scale IQ, verbal and performance subtests.

## The verbal tests

These are given and answered orally to measure verbal ability. The subtests usually include:

- defining words in ascending order of difficulty
- explaining similarities represented by common objects or concepts
- general knowledge questions and understanding of social practices
- mental arithmetic

### Digit span subtest

A dyslexic may be quite articulate and show particular abilities in abstract thinking. However, a good sign of a specific learning difference is the result of the digit span subtest. This requires the child to recall a sequence of numbers and letters, and also in reverse order, immediately after hearing them.

You will probably be aware that the short-term memory is an area of weakness for a dyslexic, and this measure for short-term auditory memory will be a challenge and a solid indicator of dyslexia.

## The performance tests

These are tests given and answered by looking at, drawing or manipulating pictures. The subtests usually include:

- completing a picture, the power of observation
- block design – duplicating a pattern using coloured bricks, measuring spatial reasoning
- matrix reasoning – selecting a missing portion from an analysis of features

Dyslexics often do particularly well in these subtests and can quite enjoy the visual-spatial block designs. For once a test is relatively easy for them and they can excel.

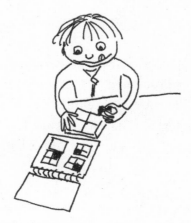

The indicators for dyslexia in these performance tests are those that measure processing speed and short-term visual memory.

Coding subtest
This requires a series of symbols to be transcribed within a specific time period, usually two minutes.

Symbol search subtest
This requires scanning a series of visual symbols and finding matches of specific targets within the set time period. If there are discrepancies in the results of these subtests compared to overall ability, then dyslexia could be signposted.

**The test results**
IQ scores are calculated according to what may be expected of a child, depending on the child's age. If children complete items in a test beyond

what is expected for an average child of their age, then ability will be described as high average (usually scored as an IQ between 110-119), high or superior (usually scored as an IQ between 120-129) and exceptionally high (130+). People with dyslexia are often in the average and high average range.

However, it is best not to be too focused on these scores. There will be some ability strengths to point out to your child, but there will also be weaknesses that you do not want to emphasize. The most important information in the report, and its main 'power' for you as the advocate for your child, is <u>the percentiles and recommendations.</u>

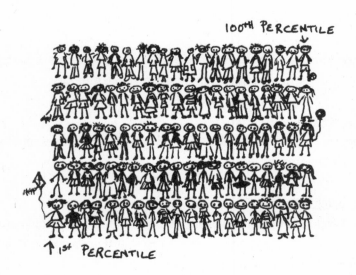

Percentiles show where a child is in a typical group of 100 children of the same age in terms of achievement on a particular task. For example, a child placed at the 90th percentile in mathematical skills will be achieving as well as or better than 90 per cent of her peers; she will be in the top 10 per cent. A result of around the 50th percentile will show a good, solid average within the group. Areas of weakness could produce a result between the 1st and 10th percentile, particularly in areas of reading and spelling. This child would be performing below 90 per cent of her peers.

Don't despair; this could prove very valuable for any extra support in school and for the state exams.

The report may include scaled scores as another scoring system within each subtest. These are scored on a scale from 1-19, where 8-12 is the average range.

Coding and Digit Span are likely to be areas of weakness with scores around 6, while Vocabulary and Block Design could be in the above-average range with scores around 16.

Dyslexic children often excel in certain subtests, showing a scaled score of 13 and above, and clear strengths in either verbal ability or non-verbal ability. Such information should be very useful for teaching methods, and for capitalizing on a dyslexic child's strengths in support of any assessed weaknesses. Good progress can be made with this significant insight into how an individual child prefers to learn. And, of course, this has a huge consequence for self-confidence.

However, all this is dependent on teachers and the school taking the details of the report on board and implementing recommended approaches. (See Chapter 11 for your role in this.)

## Summary and recommendations

The final part of the report is the most important section for you, your child and the school. Through working in partnership with the school, you can offer the emotional and practical support at home, while the school implements the educational plan.

The psychologist will recommend learning support or resource hours in school, and possibly further referral to other specialists, such as an Occupational Therapist, to pursue a possible co-existing difficulty. Often dyspraxia, dysgraphia or Irlen Syndrome are present with dyslexia. (See the Appendix for further information on these particular areas.)

Follow the recommendations, take a look at the recommended websites, apps and so on. This is your focus once you have that report. It is your plan of action. Therefore an educational psychologist's report is very advantageous if used effectively. It assists in giving direction on how best to support your child. It outlines supportive measures to enable your child to flourish and to put a constructive educational plan in place.

## You Have the Report . . . What Next?

You have a 'diagnosis' of a specific learning disability or difficulty / dyslexia / dyslexic tendencies (depending on how the professional prefers to phrase the results in the report). The best advice would be from parents and children who have already been through this whole experience. The first thing to remember is: **don't panic**!

> 'Once parents get a diagnosis, don't panic. They should look on this as the first step in getting the important help for their child. Approach the school and see what they can offer the child. There is lots of help and there are lots of kids with dyslexia.'
>
> Therese, parent

### Arrange meetings with the school

Go to the school armed with the report and plenty of copies to be given to the Principal, class teacher, resource teacher, and anyone else who works with your child. You cannot guarantee that the report will be circulated on your behalf, so it is advisable to hand over the report physically at your meetings.

Communication at primary school may be a little easier than at secondary school, where there will be many subject teachers who will not be aware of all the specific learning differences across their classes.

> 'Once there is a diagnosis, work with the report and the resource teacher and class teacher to make a plan of action. In secondary school, this is a lot harder as there are many teachers and some may not be as understanding.'
>
> Maria, parent

> 'The teachers didn't click why I was finding it difficult. My parents went to the Principal to explain I might not be able to do as well as the rest of them. Explaining to people who are helping is the best they can do.'
>
> Aoife, 13

## Find out what you can about dyslexia

Take it upon yourself to find out as much as you can about dyslexia – books, the Internet, other parents and so on.

> 'The problem with dyslexia is "Where do I start?" . . . and, in my case, it was not at school.'
>
> Margaret, parent

> 'I would suggest read up and become familiar with everything you can find about dyslexia. The information online, the support groups, the support teachers, and talk it over with your child and know about

it. It explains a lot! And it helps to know that the child is not "lazy", "stupid", "doing it on purpose", all those unhelpful and completely incorrect statements.'

Niamh, parent

'Every child is different. Ask people you know who have a son or daughter who is dyslexic, research it, get your own understanding. Just get an in-depth opinion from parents, children, teachers. Go to a talk. Ask your child what it is, what do they find difficult? You can't stress enough that parents need to know exactly what is going on. Even if they can't experience it themselves, they need to know what it is to that child. If you have other children with it, they are all going to be different. Ask your child!'

Tadhg's excellent advice as a dyslexic teenager

## Join your local association
- become a member of the national and local organization
- go to meetings
- join any support groups
- attend parent talks on assistive technology
- join workshops available for children with dyslexia

'Go to your local dyslexia association meetings. Talk to other parents. Find a tutor outside of school who can help your child to learn and give advice on technology.'

Margaret, parent

'I joined the Dyslexia Association and my son joined the weekly workshops. He met children of his own age with learning issues that were similar to his and it was a very positive experience for him. It seemed to make him more relaxed about it knowing that he wasn't on his own.'

Mary, parent

## Get outside specialist support

Sometimes, parents (and their children) feel they are not receiving the support their child requires or deserves through the general education system, and decide to look elsewhere for specialist tuition with a private tutor. If you can afford private tuition then go for it. But make sure you find a tutor specifically trained in dyslexia.

> 'Find a good dyslexia teacher.'
>
> Dolores, parent

There are many individuals working in learning support who are known as 'special needs' tutors. But as you now know, people with dyslexia are not in the 'special needs' category, they are just individuals who process information differently, and you need a tutor who recognizes that. Your local association should have a list of dyslexia-trained tutors in your area but, of course, the best advice is to seek out recommendations from other parents. Word of mouth and the parent network is always the best option for finding a good tutor.

> 'Be positive about it, be there, be supportive. It's not a scary thing. Get outside help from someone who knows what they're talking about. You need someone who is fully aware and actually trained.'
>
> Katie, a dyslexic student's advice

## Keep being an advocate for your child (see Chapter 11)

No one is going to care as much about your child's school experience and self-esteem as you, so keep reminding those who work with your child of the support infrastructure they promised but has maybe fallen by the wayside a little. You can't be a teacher at home, you are the emotional support, but you can certainly remind others to take heed of the recommendations in the psychologist's report, whether it is to do with the full resource hours at primary school or exam support at secondary school. Be persistent.

> 'Get the resource in place in school, get on to teachers and do out a plan. Keep on top of the plan! Join the national association. If you can afford it, look to someone to help with learning through dyslexia.'
>
> Elmarie, a parent's advice

## Talk to your child

This final step is most important, and is actually your first move, as well as talking with your child throughout the entire process. See the next chapter on how to explain dyslexia to your child and deal with any feelings that arise.

### Takeaways from Chapter 3

- don't delay in looking for professional advice
- understand the report and follow up on any recommendations
- liaise with school for support and find outside support systems and interventions
- don't panic, don't feel bad

## CHAPTER FOUR

# How to Talk about Dyslexia and Handle Feelings

'I actually felt pretty happy being dyslexic and happy to have dyslexia. I thought it was a rare thing, I must be pretty lucky to have this. I was happy to find more people struggle just like me, and it is not a bad thing at all. I just told my whole class because I was so excited! What gave me confidence was talking to my mum and just me being me.'

Sean, 13

## The Importance of Talking with Your Child

This chapter focuses on the importance of talking everything through with your child. It looks at the dominant feelings for young and older children, and how you can help by:

- being open and honest
- being positive and encouraging
- educating others

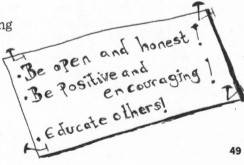

This chapter avoids the word 'diagnosis' or 'diagnosed', which is difficult to do when discussing a perceived disability. The word 'diagnosis' is loaded with negative connotations – of an illness, an affliction, a disability. You don't want your child to feel that dyslexia is any of these things, so try to avoid the use of any references such as 'being diagnosed with dyslexia', 'after diagnosis' and so on. It does not help your child's self-image nor your household's attitude to dyslexia.

You also now have to educate others on how people with dyslexia do not see it as a 'diagnosis' to be ashamed of or pitied, but it is part of who they are and their way of seeing the world. As soon as you are aware you are a parent of a dyslexic child, change the language around it and correct others!

> **CASE STUDY**
>
> **KATIE, ON THE LANGUAGE OF BEING 'DIAGNOSED' AT 10**
>
> 'I still have a weird thing around the word "diagnosed" with dyslexia. To me that was a medical term – you've been "diagnosed" with dyslexia. I felt like I was sick, like I had just had a blood test and got something wrong with me. I didn't feel relief at all.
>
> The language around dyslexia as if it's a sickness can be very daunting for someone that age. It took a long while to get over this whole "diagnosis". I felt different about school after my "diagnosis". I have to get better . . . I have to be normal, get healthy.
>
> As I got older, I realized it wasn't a diagnosis.'

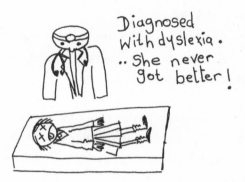

Use other phrases, for example: we 'recognized', 'discovered' or 'spotted' dyslexia; it was a 'realization', 'a revelation', 'a lightbulb moment when we found out'.

## Telling Your Child about Dyslexia

You will have a mixture of feelings once your child's dyslexia has been confirmed. It could be quite a shock, you may feel angry at the school for not spotting it sooner, and blame yourself for not doing something about it earlier. If you have dyslexia as well, you may feel guilt that you have passed it on to your child. And if your memories of school were painful because of your own dyslexia, you may be fearful that your child will have a similar experience. You may feel sad and worry about your child's future. You might overreact!

### Stay calm

Find out as much as you can about dyslexia and take a matter-of-fact approach. Remember that the way your child reacts to dyslexia will be greatly influenced by your attitude to it.

> 'It could be quite emotional for a small kid . . . make sure they don't feel a freak and a bigger deal than it is.'
>
> Niamh's advice

## Be positive about the 'label'

It is crucial that you show a positive and confident attitude from the start. Remember, dyslexia is not a disability; it is not something to be embarrassed by or ashamed of.

Your child will be sensitive to any negative feelings around the report and a dyslexia 'label'. There are some widely held attitudes that children should not be labelled. Schools avoid definitive labels, and some educational psychologists avoid the word 'dyslexia'. Unfortunately, such approaches can add to the idea of shame and struggle around this learning difference. Trust that those who work closely with parents and children with dyslexia overwhelmingly prefer to have the 'label' dyslexia written in the report and recognized by the school. Parents then feel more confident in their position to make sure their children receive all the support they deserve.

> 'Parents need to be strong for their child . . . they need to portray the good sides to having dyslexia and take away any negativity.'
>
> Luke's advice

## Be open

Be honest from the start, talk about it freely. Go through the report with your child; it is about him, after all, and no one else.

> 'The educational psychologist's report is reading something very personal to you in a very impersonal way. You are looking at how deficient you are in certain aspects, so it can be quite disheartening. But I found it good to read it myself. If the child is curious about what is in the actual document, sit down and read parts of it with them. When it's about them, they should be involved in it regardless. Just make sure they are emotionally supported.'
>
> Mike's advice

## Valuable advice from parents of children with dyslexia

'Talk about dyslexia straight away – be open with your child, tell them exactly what is going on, the children know themselves.'

Brenda

'Honesty is the best way to avoid unnecessary negative experiences. Sit down and explain what the report says. Usually, the child is relieved to know that there is a reason that they are finding things difficult. Give them examples of famous people who are also dyslexic. Explain that they will have strengths in other areas and will just have to approach learning in a different way and work that little bit harder.'

Therese

'Emphasize other talents. Consider dyslexia as a positive aspect . . . emphasize that doors are not closed!'

Françoise

'Talk openly at home about the advantages and disadvantages of dyslexia. Acknowledge frustrations and listen to the child, help them develop their own coping skills.'

Dolores

'Introduce other dyslexics, especially highlight family members. A bit of humour can defuse things, too.'

Lisa

## Knowing is always better than not knowing

You and your family members will need to learn more about dyslexia, but essentially your relationship with your child has not changed. This is just a confirmation that she learns differently, and it has nothing to do with her intelligence. Knowledge will give you confidence in combatting any negative reactions and ignorance coming from others less knowledgeable. Fortunately, attitudes are changing, and talking about dyslexia is becoming more open and positive. You may have noticed some celebrities and sports personalities have been talking about their dyslexia all of a sudden. You must encourage acceptance in society, change the negative language around dyslexia, and start to educate others about this different way of thinking.

> 'If you are a parent of someone with dyslexia, don't think of it as a deformity. You may have a genius on your hands!'[1]
>
> Benjamin Zephaniah, poet

## Talking to Younger Children

Translate the language of the report to a language level more suitable for young children. Don't hide it; there is no reason to do this, and often children can feel relief that they now have an answer for their difficulties, that they're not stupid after all.

> 'It was a HUGE relief. Tell them because it is such a relief to know there is a reason for all this. She was relieved because there's a piece of paper now that says, "I'm really smart."'
>
> Danielle, parent

> 'Emotionally, there was a sense of relief because once we started putting things in place to help him, he flourished all the way.'
>
> Kate, parent

Make sure you explain that dyslexia is very common and there are probably some other dyslexics in their class.

......................................
It is important that they know they are not alone.
......................................

Do some research and point out all the famous actors, writers, musicians, sports people, scientists, artists, inventors and entrepreneurs with dyslexia. Draw attention to their own abilities and strengths, reassure them on areas that they are particularly good at.

'I would advise a parent to just speak to the child. Talk about how it is so common, so many famous people are dyslexic, point out the various celebrities. This can help to make them see it's not that "big a deal", and that it doesn't hold people back. I think they can relate when you mention somebody famous, especially if it's someone they like or admire. It is just a "thing" and not the whole of the person, and that they just learn differently to others, and so what? It doesn't define them as a person.'

Niamh, parent

'It's more common than you ever could imagine . . . you're not alone. And there are ways to accelerate your skills.'[2]

Steven Spielberg, film director

## Be sensitive

You may need to apologize for not understanding those struggles during stressful, protracted homework sessions, and so promise to learn more about your child's learning style from now on.

'It is up to the parents to accept it and inform themselves and go with it.'

Uwe, parent

'No child wants to be different. Be sensitive at home to what they need to tell you. Listen and you will pick up what is difficult for them.'

Liz, parent

'Encourage them all the time. Give them a break! They are not stupid, they just learn differently. Tell them the world is run by dyslexics, show them who these people are from the Internet. It is a unique attribute that they can give to the world. It can help them, not hinder them.'

Elmarie, parent

## Personal stories from children who found out they were dyslexic at a young age

'I used to love the Pirates of the Caribbean movies when I was little, and to know they all had dyslexia was good.'

Helena, 12

'I felt better, that I wasn't just bad at reading.'

Anna, 9

'I felt fine about it! I didn't know what it was! I have dyslexia, no big deal.'

Luca, 10

'"Oh, I have dyslexia and you don't!" I thought it was something good. I'd say to my friend, "Do you have dyslexia?" And she'd say, "No," and I'd say, "I have it!"'

Caoimhe, 14

'I felt relief – relieved I was not stupid, and a little bit scared I'd be put in a different class from my friends, and I felt I had a secret and I had to protect my secret. Sometimes, I would identify other dyslexics in the playground – oh, I've figured out their secret!'

Niamh, remembering primary school

'You're not stupid! You're clever in your own way, so keep your head up high and don't let anyone tell you you're stupid . . . just say, "I'm not!"'

Céire, 12

As these memories show, the child can, in fact, react more positively and be more relaxed and accepting than the parent! The most common feeling is relief. However, it can be complex at times when your child is processing this new-found discovery, and it becomes more challenging the older the child is.

Be prepared to talk through your child's learning difference at various times over the years. And if you can get a specialist to discuss your child's particular strengths and weaknesses with him, then that would be ideal.

## Talking to Teenage Children

### Mixed feelings

Although there appears to be more awareness of dyslexia in present times, there continues to be a substantial number of children who are not identified as dyslexic until secondary school. At this stage, they may have already experienced a fair amount of failure and a loss of confidence and self-belief. The school may have failed to recognize or accept the dyslexia, and emotional and behavioural problems may have emerged, partly due to those feelings of uselessness and failure.
The teenage child may react badly to this discovery, angry that it wasn't dealt with earlier by their parents or school. They may refuse to accept it or any support strategies offered.

Teenagers don't usually want to be seen as 'different'. They are sensitive to how they are being regarded by their peers. Any self-consciousness felt from suddenly being 'diagnosed' with a 'disability' can be excruciating for the teenager. No wonder that the older you are, the more complex this discovery can be.

## The mixed feelings about a dyslexia 'diagnosis' as a teenager

'I didn't really know what it was. I was a bit confused and upset by it. I was embarrassed and I didn't want to talk about it.'

Aoibhinn

'I don't think I felt much better, if I'm honest. Dyslexia seems to have some sort of label that people don't understand.'

Emma

'I didn't want to have dyslexia at first, I felt so stupid. I felt it was a bad thing, but then it's not, it's grand. I learnt a lot of people have it, it's not bad.'

Abbie

'I don't care if I'm different. If anything I was telling people, so if I made a stupid mistake . . . "Oh, he's dyslexic, that's OK." I'd use it to get sympathy points!'

Tadhg

'When it did click that I have dyslexia, it all suddenly made sense. I felt like a weight had been lifted off my shoulders, but I was also so frustrated with myself for having it, while my sisters, friends and family didn't. I thought it was totally unfair. I felt angry towards the world because it meant that I had to, and still do, work so much harder than everyone else and, for the most part, not get any recognition for it.'

Nicola

'After being diagnosed, at first I felt upset and angry, but as my time grew with dyslexia, I felt better about myself. I wasn't worried about telling people because I knew they would understand and support me.'

Claire

## What you can do to help

In order to help your teenager cope with the knowledge that he is dyslexic, it's important to:

- reassure
- encourage and support
- remember there is absolutely nothing 'wrong'
- educate yourself and others, be positive, be open

They need to feel that they do have ability and that they can succeed. The teenage dyslexics should go through their own report (it is about them after all). The breakdown of subtests in the report should be invaluable in pointing out strengths and abilities. They need to know that they can succeed, and that this is not a 'disability' nor a barrier to success. Parents can be supportive by talking about it as a learning difference that does not have to affect school success, and discussing it in a casual situation like a car journey can take the stress out of the conversation.

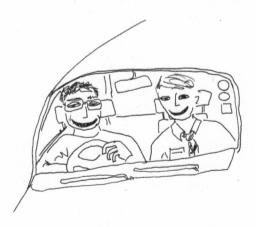

At the same time, parents must not allow dyslexia to be used as an excuse not to try, nor allow the school to stop challenging the dyslexic teenager. Dyslexics are well able, and giving up on them or allowing them to make do with unchallenging work is doing them a disservice and feeding into a poor self-image. Encouraging strengths and interests outside of school is also crucial for the reluctant teenage dyslexic.

> 'I think support is the word, you can't put enough emphasis on support. He had a good relationship with everybody who helped him and I think that helped with his confidence.'
>
> Kate, parent

## And finally – leave them to it!

Once you have passed on all you have found out about dyslexia and helped your older child to pursue her strengths and abilities, you can then leave her to explore and accept her different way of thinking and learning in whatever way suits her. Know how to explain dyslexia to others, but also know when to step back and allow your teenage dyslexic to express her dyslexia as she wishes.

> 'I used to get cross when my mum told people.'
>
> Emily, 18

> 'Let them tell people when they're ready. It's up to me who I tell.'
>
> Aoibhinn's advice, 14

Make sure you leave it up to your child to tell others. It isn't your story, it is her story and she owns her dyslexia.

Older children can have the confidence instilled by their parents and others to then talk to teachers themselves about their dyslexia and what they need in school. It is up to them to tell their friends or not.

## Work on a tag-line to help explain dyslexia to others

Being confident, and wanting to educate others, will reflect a successful outcome in the whole process; from 'diagnosis' to then implementing support strategies. Confidence in a clear definition of dyslexia will immediately give the listener a positive view of this perceived 'disability', and help transform the dominant image of dyslexia.

Encourage a 'tag-line' – a short catchy definition of dyslexia to tell others. For example: 'It is a learning difference, just a different way of processing information'; 'It just means you learn differently, it can take a little longer to take in information'; 'It is not a disability, it is a creative strength, a unique way of looking at the world'.

### Takeaways from Chapter 4

- be open and honest from the start
- be positive in your language around the word
- educate yourself so you can educate others
- allow your child to own it

## CHAPTER FIVE

# Helping with Reading

'Reading was difficult, everyone else would be finished reading the page and I would be only halfway through and I would say I am done, too, but I never was. It made me feel disappointed with myself because I felt I was the only one.'

Claire, 14, remembering her primary school experiences with reading

## Helping Your Child to Become a Confident Reader

This chapter will explore how you can help your child deal with the challenges of becoming a confident reader. It looks at specific stages in learning to read and its difficulties from the early years to secondary school by providing:

- ideas to support the initial stages of learning to read
- tools to encourage comprehension and fluency
- ways to make reading more fun
- solutions for the older reader

The process of reading is a learnt skill that can take some of us longer than others to master, but eventually it is something most of us do automatically. However, if we break down the skills involved, we can see the challenges for the dyslexic. There are three aspects of reading for the dyslexic to master:

1. <u>decoding words</u> – the ability to recognize letters and their corresponding sounds, being able to sound out a word
2. <u>comprehension</u> – ability to understand what we read
3. <u>fluency</u> – ability to read quickly and accurately with flow

Dyslexic individuals can struggle with any or all of these areas on their path to being a good reader.

Although references will be made to primary and secondary school experiences, the difficulties with phonics, comprehension and fluency can be experienced at any age, and the practical advice will be relevant at any stage in a dyslexic individual's aim to become an accomplished reader.

In the past, before we had the understanding of dyslexia that we have now, it was a 'disability' referred to as 'word blindness'. This signifies to us that the acquisition of word attack skills and reading fluency has always been the most significant (and sometimes seen as the only) issue for people with dyslexia.

So much emphasis is placed on reading from an early age. A difficulty with reading is often the first point in a child's learning where parents sense there is a 'problem'. It must be mentioned here that children develop at different rates, so where one child may be ready to read at four years old, another may not 'click' with reading until much later. If your child has tried and failed at reading by seven years old or older, it is worth looking into the possibility of a learning difference. Early identification is undoubtedly very important for children with dyslexia.

Without the right intervention early on, a child may drop further and further behind her peers as reading becomes more challenging. This emphasis from the start of her school career to accomplish word reading becomes a burden, often leaving her feeling stupid, inadequate or somehow deficient. Your dyslexic child is quite possibly very articulate and creative, with a good understanding of challenging concepts, yet has enormous difficulty when faced with the written word. This exposure of poor reading ability is so demoralizing for the intelligent, very aware dyslexic child.

Reading is essential. Any struggle with reading is emotive, exposing and dispiriting. Here are dyslexic teenagers remembering their experiences of reading at primary school:

> 'I wouldn't be able to grasp stuff because I'd skip a word I couldn't get. I just thought I was slow.'
>
> Sarah, 15

> 'I remember a cloze test comprehension when I had to choose the right word. I was only halfway through. I got so upset, I could not do it. I still remember that, I was only about eight years old.'
>
> Jennifer, 18

> 'I remember everyone else was flying through their box of words to learn, but I was one of the last people because I'd keep forgetting them. I'd try reading over them but I couldn't understand why I was one of the only ones not getting them right.'
>
> Aoife, 13

> 'I'd still be on a baby book when everyone was reading big books. I was getting annoyed – why can't I read fast like them?'
>
> Abbie, 14

Success or failure in reading can be extremely emotive, creating anxiety for children as well as parents, who may recognize in their child their own struggles with reading in school.

You can't perform miracles; your child may never be a fluent reader or a book lover, but you know there are some things you can do to help along the way and encourage any progress, however small each step may be. And, of course, we are very fortunate now compared to possibly your own struggles at school, as your child has the advantages of technology – a huge boost, particularly for the access and assimilation of knowledge.

So to help with supporting your child on those first steps to becoming a confident reader, here are a series of strategies that will make a positive difference.

## Letter Sounds, Decoding Words and 'Phonological Awareness'

There is no harm in knowing the more formal phrases used by teachers and educational psychologists. A common official phrase used to evaluate a dyslexic's reading ability is 'poor grapheme-to-phoneme decoding skills'. If teachers and other professionals refer to 'graphemes' and 'phonemes' you now know that they are referencing the letter name or combination of letters (grapheme) and corresponding sound (phoneme). For example: the letters 'ph' make an 'f' sound. Knowledge is power and, as an advocate for your child, you want to be on top of what the professionals are talking about.

Reading is first the decoding of symbols. We have to translate symbols from the page into sounds, and these sounds then need to be combined to make a meaningful word.

For reading accuracy the child must:

- recognize the letter
- match the correct sound to the letter (or letter blend like 'ch', 'ph' or vowel combination like 'ai', 'ea', 'oa')

- see the letters in the correct sequence
- say the letters in the correct sequence
- remember and recognize them again next time

When we break down the beginnings of reading, we can see the work the dyslexic child must undertake to be able to read.

> 'Getting every word right in a sentence, it makes me feel cross not getting it right.'
>
> Anna, 9

Becoming a skilled reader means being able to decode words. Children with dyslexia have problems with 'phonological awareness' and 'phonological development' – the learning of sounds and their corresponding symbols to progress to reading fluency. Initially, the challenge for the dyslexic child is the ability to use phonological awareness to decipher unfamiliar words and therefore get on the path to becoming a more independent reader.

### How you can help your dyslexic child to recognize and decode words

As emphasized throughout this guide, and most significantly in Chapters 5-10, multi-sensory learning and capitalizing on the right-brained creative strength of the dyslexic individual is the way to go forward with any learning challenges.

Reading is the decoding of words – letters have names, sounds, shapes and a feel (when written). The aim is to help your child to see, hear and feel letters and sounds. A multi-sensory approach is very beneficial for the dyslexic with a weak working memory. Learning through several learning channels at once will help the dyslexic tap into his preferred learning style.

If there is a history of dyslexia in the family then there is no harm in starting phonic awareness at home at an early age. There is plenty of commercially available material out there to help with phonics, such as www.toe-by-toe.co.uk and www.wordshark.co.uk.

Some ideas:

- find rhyming words in songs and books
- clap the syllables of words
- encourage tracing letters in sand, on the table or in large arm movements in the air
- encourage making letters with Play-Doh or pipe-cleaners
- find commercially available material with step-by-step phonic practice, such as Toe-by-Toe or Synthetic Phonics

Some of the phonic material out there can be an incredibly dry read and rarely enjoyed by parent or child. So it is important also to find some reading activities that you will both enjoy, will not put too much pressure on your child but will challenge a little.

Keep a look out for games you can play that will encourage letter and word recognition – play card games such as 'syllable snap' or 'pairs' and 'phonic dominoes', quiz games that require reading information aloud, and computer games such as 'Wordshark'. Lots of varied, small activities will help your child become more aware of phonics and how to decode unfamiliar words.

'Sounding the words out helps – picking out small bits in words.'

Anna, 9

> 'Once I taught him the phonics, he was fine. The difference was just unbelievable once he got it, once we got back to basics and taught him the phonics of the alphabet.'
>
> Yvonne, parent

Of course, not all words will neatly fit this breaking down to corresponding sounds, with their silent letters and inexplicable exceptions to the rule. There is no real solution for these idiosyncrasies to the English language other than practising and building a sight vocabulary. Reading together and playing word games will help.

## Comprehending What is Being Read

Comprehension is the ability to get meaning from what we have read. A dyslexic child concentrating all his efforts on the decoding of each word in a sentence may lose sight of the meaning of what he is trying to read. He may have to go over the sentence or paragraph several times to gain full comprehension. Alternatively, he may avoid reading and find clever tactics to give the impression he can read and comprehend the words on the page.

Clues that he is using clever tactics to hide the fact he is not actually reading:

- relying on pictures and contextual clues
- memorizing the story from hearing it several times

> 'One of my earliest memories I have is of being caught out with a simple reading book in primary school. The book was very simple with one sentence per page filled out with large pictures. I had developed a coping strategy of remembering what the other children were reading and, in turn, repeating this for my turn.'
>
> Luke, engineer

Reading difficulties will manifest initially with the actual mechanics of reading, and while the recognition of individual words may be well practised, there will quite probably remain a difficulty with comprehension. A child's good work on the sounding out of words does not help with extracting meaning from the page.

> 'I'd skip a few lines. I'd see the word and just assume the wrong word and continue reading but it wouldn't make any sense.'
>
> Aoibhinn, 14, remembering her early years

So how can you help your child to understand what he is reading, and hopefully instil an enjoyment in connecting the words with an overall meaning, a tale, or a gripping story?

The first point is – you cannot be a teacher at home! You are the parent and not part of the torment of the reading scheme at school. What you can do is encourage skills in comprehension – model good reading for your child, engage your child in reading with you, and encourage games and activities that include the need for comprehending what is being read.

Here are some ideas:

- Cut up cartoon strips (from comics like the ever-popular <u>Beano</u> and the more contemporary and very popular Manga comics). Mix them up and get your child to arrange the sections to recreate the story in the correct sequence.
- Find appropriate games with a demand for reading comprehension, such as trivia quizzes.
- Have the subtitles option on your screen for favourite TV shows and cartoons.
- Read together – be engaged together, asking questions, discussing the content.

'As soon as she saw Manga cartoons, she wanted to read them! And she watches these cartoons with English subtitles. She has to read at speed and glean some information from it – so she wants to actively read them.'

Danielle, parent

## Achieving Reading Fluency

'It was extremely hard in primary school. It took me a very long time to develop any sort of flow in my reading without being stuck at words.'

Ben, graduate

### Paired reading

Paired reading is reading aloud with a fluent reader. It is one of the best ways to improve fluency.

'Weekends were an opportunity to focus on reading. Reading every second paragraph – I loved that.'

Mike, remembering paired reading with his parents

It is important to model good reading from an early age, and fluency will grow through the shared activity of paired reading. Hearing a fluent reader who models correct pronunciation and use of punctuation is invaluable, as well as giving an opportunity to explain the meaning of words and discuss the content of the book.

'I couldn't read. I didn't really know I couldn't read. I'd read across the page, from page to page, I didn't know how to read.'

Caoimhe, 14, remembering her early primary years

And remember, reading can be a stressful experience for a dyslexic so be careful how you approach reading together.

## How to approach paired reading

- Have a calm, relaxed, quiet space nowhere near the usual homework space
- Your child chooses the book to read (although you will guide them towards a suitable level, not too easy or too challenging)
- Sit side by side
- Take it in turns to read a paragraph or a page, depending on ability
- Initially you could read the paragraphs together, your own voice getting softer as your child gains confidence
- Encourage your child to follow the words on the page when it is your turn to read
- If your child stumbles over a word DO NOT be a teacher and break down the sounds of the word; just say the word – keep the fluency going, and your child then repeats the word and carries on
- Give a few seconds to allow your child to attempt a difficult word, keep the flow and enjoyment, otherwise labouring over the challenges will make it a very negative experience
- Set a comfortable pace for you both
- Encourage and praise
- Do paired reading together every day if you can or at least three days a week, for about fifteen minutes
- Enjoy having valuable time together, just the two of you

'I loved paired reading. I did it with my mum all the time. When you concentrate so much on reading and getting all the words right you can sometimes miss the message of the text. It was really good to listen to someone and someone you actually trust and you can fully go "OK, I'm going to read this to you now, ignore my mistakes, don't judge me." I was completely open and confident. The relaxed environment you are reading in really helps.'

Katie, remembering paired reading at home

Reading improves with practice. So when you aren't doing some paired reading with your child, rope in another family member, a grandparent, uncle or aunt, someone your child feels comfortable to make mistakes with when reading aloud.

## Other ideas for reading fluency

Reading to a pet – if you have a dog, you are in the fortunate position of giving your child an advantage in reading. Research has shown that reading to your pet dog can improve reading fluency by up to 20 per cent, according to anecdotal evidence from parents, teachers, librarians and academic research at the University of California in 2010. The presence of a dog – non-judgemental and calming for the unconfident reader – can be a valuable experience as they sit together, just the two of them. And if you have other types of pets, such as a cat, it's still worth trying, although dogs are naturally inclined to show some interest and will probably enjoy the opportunity of contact that a reading session will offer.

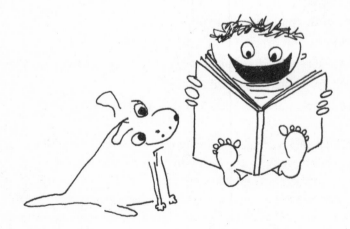

Encourage their own choice of reading material – make sure your child takes his first step into reading fluency by choosing the material himself, whatever engages him, whether it is a fiction book, a science or history book, a comic, a website. Anything that truly engages him will always be better than something that seems to be more appropriate but doesn't capture his attention.

<u>Using a marker to support reading</u> – it is OK to use a bookmarker, card, pen or ruler to keep the eye on the line being read, especially when tired. Instead of having the marker below the line, place it above the line being read, so you are not obscuring what is to come and there is more flow and comprehension.

<u>The advantages of technology to help fluency</u> – audiobooks are a great way to improve fluency. You can download thousands of books read by authors and actors on to your device. Your child can then experience a good model of fluency and expression, and be exposed to wider vocabulary.

A text-to-speech option is available with most computers and e-readers, and can often be adjusted to different speeds. At a reasonable pace, the printed text can be followed at the same time, thus encouraging fluency. Kindles, for example, have a text-to-speech feature and can change print size and colour background.

> 'The Kindle usually helps me – you can make the print bigger. If you are struggling with a word you can look at it up close, you can't do that with a book.'
>
> Aoife, 13

> 'Read them books and they will understand that knowledge is in there and that even if they never learn to read in a flowing way, they will find a way to get that knowledge out. They will read it or find someone to read it or a computer program to read it to them or a video to say it to them.'
>
> Cathal, parent

## The Pleasure of Reading

'I've always wanted to enjoy reading, I've always envied that. I'd love to be able to just sit down and read a book.'

Tadhg, 15

It can be a huge challenge to transform a child's misgivings and aversion to reading for pleasure. Be prepared for, and be accepting, if your child does not become an avid reader – not everyone will be. But there are certain things you can do – and not do – to help your dyslexic child find an appreciation of reading as a way of gaining knowledge and entertainment. And you never know, she may find the book that ignites her interest and a love of reading in her own time.

### How you can help to make reading more fun

There is a huge risk that children with dyslexia, and adults, see reading as a way of receiving information and learning rather than a pleasure in itself. Parents can really help to establish reading as a pleasure for young children and to see it as a way of opening their minds to different worlds.

Don't be anxious about reading. You may have experienced reading difficulties yourself at her age, and associated anxiety and failure around learning to read. And yet now you have to be the positive one about reading, and encourage your child to feel the opposite of how you felt at her age. It can be a stressful time for the parent as well as the child.

Here are some ideas to help your child enjoy reading:

- It is always good to read to children, to talk about stories, to look at pictures and to ask questions.
- In the early years, reading books with rhythm and rhyme, such as <u>Dr Seuss</u> books, help to develop fluency and enjoyment.

- Audiobooks – it may be more conducive for you to enjoy listening to books together, finding audiobooks and other options. Listening to stories will encourage pleasure in the content of a book and hopefully a desire to find out more. A popular series of books can be listened to on car journeys and encouraged to be read independently.
- This is important – <u>don't force books on to your child</u>, and don't think that reading more will 'cure' the dyslexic difficulties with reading.

> 'She just won't pick up a book! We have books around and hope she will pick one up. I buy her tons of books, and she's not a bit interested.'
>
> Danielle, parent

Encourage any material that will capture your child's interest or imagination:

- the non-fiction books and magazines that connect with a hobby or interest
- the genre that grips the child
- a particular author, a book series, where a child gains momentum moving from one finished book to the next in the series

> 'I found a certain type of book I wanted to read. As I enjoy History, I connected with stories about war and history.'
>
> Sean, 13

Finding a favourite author and book series is the key to success. Discovering a particular author, genre and series of books is what will really instil a pleasure in reading into the dyslexic individual. This can only happen somehow organically, possibly through peers being big readers of popular authors, such as David Walliams, Roald Dahl, J. K. Rowling.

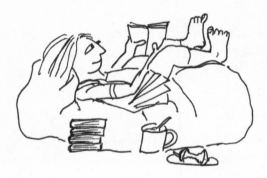

'I used to hate reading. Only when I found a book myself and then I loved reading and I just couldn't stop. Everyone was reading at the time the "big reads" and I wanted to be part of it. I read the whole series (the Twilight series by Stephenie Meyer) really fast and then another series (the Gone series by Michael Grant).'

Juliette, 17, on how she became an avid reader

Remember that discovering the pleasure of reading can come at any age. Your child may not take up reading for pleasure until the teenage years, college or later.

Look out for attractive, dyslexia-friendly books. A book needs to be instantly readable. Children with dyslexia want large print, ample spacing and a suitable typeface. Encourage your child to choose a book that has appealing print, colour and pictures. She will know what appeals to her. Dyslexia-friendly material will have a better visual impact for the dyslexic child.

'Look for dyslexic-friendly books, get an iPad and download some fun word games. Let them use the Internet to look up words. Use the summer for as much fun paired reading as possible. Dyslexic kids absolutely appreciate wins. Because they have to work harder to learn to read it is all the sweeter when they have successes.'

Lisa, parent, on making learning to read accessible and fun

## Dyslexia-Friendly Books

Children with dyslexia may find the following visual aspects more appealing when choosing a book to read:

- larger print
- sans-serif-style font is easier to read (not with curly bits); for example Arial, Comic Sans and Verdana, and a point size of 12
- well-spaced text and line spacing
- colour backgrounds
- cartoons and speech bubbles
- plenty of colour and illustrations
- short paragraphs and chapters
- avoiding glossy paper and bright white

Look into the possibility of a visual perception difficulty. Your child may be experiencing sensitivity to a specific frequency and wavelength of the white light spectrum. This is known as Irlen Syndrome or Scotopic Sensitivity, a visual perception problem that affects reading.

> This is a  block of text  which contains rivers, most  people don't notice them but for a person with any  visual distortion when they are  reading it is like  a wiggly white light line  which is actually  much more apparent  than the text.  It is annoying to say  the least.  Other distortions include  glowing blobs beside text, unlike rivers  they are  not really there. Other people  see the lines of text appearing to be in  squiggly lines or to be doubled or fuzzy.

Things to look out for that could be investigated further:

- a particular preference for coloured backgrounds to pages, Kindle or computer screen
- certain physical observations when reading, such as moving closer or further away from the page, squinting, rubbing eyes, watery eyes, shielding the eyes
- complaining of headaches and tiredness, feeling nausea
- dislike of glare on the page or screen, complaining of the white pages and black print
- mentioning movement on the page, the print blurring or shaking

If any of the above is familiar to you and your child then seek a professional assessment for this visual perception difficulty. At least a third of people with reading difficulties have Irlen Syndrome or Scotopic Sensitivity, and often this visual problem co-exists with dyslexia. Don't worry, there are solutions to overcome this issue (see the Appendix for more information).

## Reading in the Secondary School Years

When children transfer from primary to secondary school, good readers flourish while poor readers may fall further behind their peers. These children who have always struggled with reading find they can't keep up with the curriculum. They are unable to follow written instructions or read the required information, so the whole of their education suffers. Confidence drains away as the challenge of reading at secondary school becomes insurmountable, possibly precipitating behavioural problems and difficult future outcomes for the dyslexic pupil. As a consequence of the failure to succeed as a fluent reader, they may never reach their potential.

It is therefore vital that you are there to help in any way you can as your dyslexic child navigates the secondary school experience.

## Challenges for older children and teenagers

- reading accuracy is affected by time pressure and stress
- having difficulty keeping their place in dense text
- having difficulty identifying the main points in a passage – scanning
- needing to read a text several times to 'digest' its contents
- can't proofread and spot their own mistakes or omissions in writing
- concentrating so much on deciphering the text they lose sight of meaning
- embarrassed and stressed by having to read aloud in class

'It was overwhelming. English was a bit of a shock! You have to make a giant leap from primary to secondary. I shied away from it because in my head it was too difficult.'

Leah, remembering her transition to secondary school

Your child may have been an OK reader in primary school, but once confronted with the dense text of textbooks in several subjects and challenging new vocabulary, difficulties with reading suddenly come to the surface. It may well be that their dyslexia isn't spotted until the pressures of reading at this higher level expose comprehension and fluency difficulties.

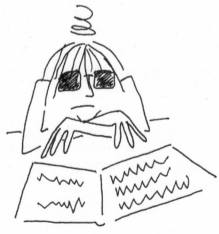

## Helping with the Challenges of Reading at School

### Make use of assistive technology

There is a wide range of ways in which dyslexic individuals can access information in our modern world. Digital texts are there for us – texts that are encoded in digital form and can be read aloud by a text-to-speech program on a computer or other device. Textbook publishers offer their publications in digital format, allowing the text-to-speech option. If they don't, then contact them and ask why. Otherwise it could be considered discrimination.

The benefits include keeping up to date with class studies, increased vocabulary and less pressure in exam studies.

> 'Pdfs of textbooks are good. If we can just get the information read to her then she can put it into her brain. It doesn't really matter how the information gets in there as long as it does.'
>
> Danielle, parent

### The dyslexic student needs technology

There are many apps recommended by professionals, schools and other parents and students that will serve your teenager well. Assistive technology, such as recorded books, scanning pens and text-to-speech software, can really enhance literary skills and fluency. The dyslexic child can have the same opportunities as others to expand his knowledge and enrich his vocabulary.

> 'I spent hours scanning in textbooks! He could hear his text as well as read it. That strengthened his memory around recognizing the word, hearing it and seeing it. He reads 400-page books now!'
>
> Uwe, parent

## You can help with homework

Your child in secondary school might appreciate you reading certain questions or pieces of text to save time and energy during homework. However, this can be a stressful time where either or both of you are impatient and liable to clash. There can be a fine line between being a useful parent and a too-involved parent! (See Chapter 9 for more on homework.)

## Encourage regular ten-minute breaks

Often your teenager with dyslexia spends hours reading textbooks over and over again, desperately trying to comprehend and absorb the information, but it just isn't going in. This causes obvious stress, anxiety and a feeling of just wanting to give up.

The effort she has to put into reading means concentration will begin to flag sooner than for a non-dyslexic student.

It is a good idea to take regular breaks and maybe switch to a less laborious task that doesn't need so much reading. Your job is to make sure she is taking frequent breaks and to encourage her to vary the ways she takes in information.

## Encourage your teenager to be an active reader

Encourage breaking down those large words in English and Science into their syllables. Make sure she has access to textbooks that she can highlight with a variety of coloured pens to support the reading skill of scanning for key points in a passage or question.

## Discuss topics studied for homework

If your teenager prefers to read aloud at home to take in information then encourage this. And listen to her discuss topics she has read, which will then help her consolidate the material in her own mind.

### Get outside help if you can

If you clash at home when it comes to homework and studies, then consider getting someone to help your child. There are specialist tutors out there if you are prepared to pay, as well as helpers who can come to the home and assist with homework.

### Be an advocate for your child when it comes to reading in class

Even though your child has strengths in verbal reasoning, imagination and so on, the effect on self-esteem of not being able to read fluently cannot be underestimated. Your job is to communicate with the school – you would be well placed to request that teachers do not ask your child to read out loud in front of others (in both primary and secondary school years).

> 'At secondary school, I really saw the difference in my reading level between myself and my peers. You'd have to read a paragraph in class in Geography or History, so then I felt exposed, felt raw.'
>
> Katie

### Look for reasonable accommodations such as a reader in the state exams

Accommodations provide a different way to gain access to knowledge. A reasonable reading speed and accuracy become essential at secondary school, especially in exam situations when a dyslexic is under pressure and a minor misreading of a sentence can have major consequences. For example, omitting the word 'not' in an exam question. Having the right and fair support at exam time is invaluable for your dyslexic child who is determined to achieve just the same as his peers. It can be the difference between grades, of getting the course he wants and the feeling he has succeeded.

Your job, and your most important role in your communication with school, is to fight for the reasonable accommodations, such as a reader. You have to be an advocate for your child (see Chapter 11).

In addition, and especially if the accommodations are not granted, you can help your teenager by getting the past exam papers for him so he can practice reading typical questions and become familiar with the exam instructions.

## CASE STUDY

### LUKE, ENGINEER, FOUND A READER INVALUABLE

'Moving to secondary school, I initially found the larger texts challenging to read and would find them tiring. This was more prevalent during exam times when texts would need to be read, processed and questions answered in a timed manner.

'I was given a reader for my exams, which really helped me to concentrate on getting the most out of my answers without worrying about how long it would take me to read the text or read the text correctly. It also meant I would not get tired reading and could use my full power to formulate answers. I actually received an A1 grade in the Leaving Certificate in higher-level English so I can guarantee it was a success.'

Learning to read and becoming an accomplished reader can be a stressful and emotional process. You may be reflecting on your own experiences. Fortunately, with the vision and determination of two dyslexic individuals – Bill Gates from Microsoft and Steve Jobs from Apple – today we can access the written word and knowledge of the world around us via the use of ever-advancing technologies.

## Home Tools to Support Reading Skills

### The primary school years

Phonics
www.toe-by-toe.co.uk
www.wordshark.co.uk
Synthetic phonics
Multi-sensory activities

Games
Syllable snap
Phonic dominoes

Comprehension
Cartoon strips
Trivia quizzes

Fluency
Paired reading
Dyslexia-friendly books
Assistive technology (text-to-speech)
Audiobooks
Pet dog or cat

### The secondary school years

Digital versions of textbooks
Coloured paper and highlighters
Past exam papers

### Takeaways from Chapter 5

- help with the early reading skills
- encourage a pleasure in reading
- find alternative ways to access the written word

## CHAPTER SIX

# Helping with Spelling

'I used to dread the spelling tests. I'd learn them so well and then the next day it would be like I hadn't learnt them at all.'

Alex, 18, remembering spelling in primary school

## Dealing with Being a Poor Speller

This chapter will provide various strategies and techniques to help your child with the challenges of spelling. It looks at specific difficulties from the early years and beyond by providing:

- ideas to tackle the sounds and patterns of words
- multi-sensory techniques for the dreaded spelling tests
- fun ways to practise the spelling of words
- solutions for the older speller

Poor spelling is perceived to be the main difficulty for people with dyslexia, while you will see across the chapters that there is far more to dyslexia than this. Nevertheless, a phonological weakness and a poor short-term memory mitigate against being a 'good speller', and this aspect of dyslexia can be a crippling issue for the dyslexic child.

If you are dyslexic, just like your child, then this will be all too familiar for you. You have got to the stage where you are accepting of the fact that you will never be a brilliant speller. But that is OK. All you can do for your child who struggles with spelling is offer help and encouragement, and also guide her to feel comfortable that although her spelling will improve, it will never be perfect.

## How you can deal with typical attitudes towards poor spellers

Unfortunately, great emphasis is still being put on spelling ability through the key stages in education. Being a good speller is applauded, a gateway to good marks and educational success, while the bad speller is condemned as careless, bound for educational failure or, worse, seen as stupid. Poor spelling can be a lifetime's embarrassment.

However, life can also be less harsh on bad spellers these days. We have technology to help us, and people are more forgiving of mistakes. Nonetheless, there is always room for improvement in other people's attitudes to dyslexia, and yet again it will be up to you as an advocate for your child to communicate to teachers that your dyslexic child cannot help those spelling errors. She does not spot her mistakes like non-dyslexic children might.

. . . . . . . . . . . . . . . . . . . . . . . . . . . . . . . . . . . . . . . . . . . . .

Remember this and remind others:
poor spelling is not an indication of low intelligence.
And good spelling is not an indication of high intelligence.

. . . . . . . . . . . . . . . . . . . . . . . . . . . . . . . . . . . . . . . . . . . . .

'The most repeating memory I have is of performing very poorly in spelling tests all through primary school. This was in contrast to excellent scores in maths tests and being classed as a "gifted" child.'

Luke, engineer

## The Challenges of Learning to Spell

Reading is given more attention in the early years, while spelling proves to be more of a struggle long-term for the dyslexic child. And no amount of reading will make you a good speller. The skill of spelling is a different process from reading. When reading, we <u>decode</u> words – we break down the letters and sounds of the word. But in spelling, we <u>encode</u> words – we do the opposite and use letter and sound knowledge to form a word. This could mean there is no visual recall for how a word is spelt in the dyslexic child's mind, but when seeing the word on the page they can recognize it and read fluently.

There are a lot of illogical letter and sound combinations in words, exceptions to rules and silent letters that you may also remember as an ordeal when you were learning to spell.

For example:

- Why do 'flour' and 'flower' sound the same but are spelt so differently?
- What is the 'l' in 'calm' for? Or the 's' in 'island'?
- Why do 'through', 'thought', 'though' and 'tough' have to be so confusing?
- Why do words have to be so long and have so many syllables?

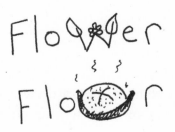

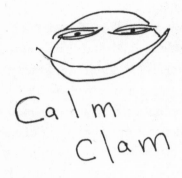

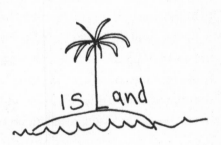

'The silent letters are difficult.'

Anna, 9

For the often logical and mathematical dyslexic brain these strange irregularities in spelling make no sense and just exasperate the otherwise very competent individual.

There are three areas in the skill of spelling that a dyslexic must work on:

1. Confidence in phonics, the sounds of letters in words. For example: 'elephant'
2. Recognition of sight words, without relying on phonics. For example: 'said'
3. An understanding of spelling rules and word families. For example: the 'magic "e"' in 'cape'

## How you can help

Support learning the spelling of words in these three areas, and you will make a difference to your child's spelling. While you are doing this, also remember and accept there is just so far you can go – you are not a teacher at home. You won't be making your child a perfect speller but you will be giving your child more confidence in how to tackle the spelling of words.

## Supporting Spelling in the Early Years

'I remember we had to vote for someone to be class leader for the week and I remember only knowing how to spell one person's name so I put that person down every week!'

> Leah, 19, remembering her early experiences at primary school

Spelling is a complex task for all young children, and even with repeated instruction in school, word attack skills will remain problematic for the dyslexic child. Weekly spelling tests are a constant ordeal for both parent and child, coupled with the sea of red pen on any free writing exercise, where on average a dyslexic pupil makes one spelling mistake per five words, while for the non-dyslexic it could be one error per thirty-five words.

'I struggled a lot with spelling when writing a story. I would get my copy book back and there would always be huge red circles around practically every single word.'

> Claire, 14, remembering creative writing exercises in primary school

### Common errors for a dyslexic child when it comes to spelling
(as well as a guide to help you spot dyslexia in your family)

- reversing letters persists – 'q'/'p', 'b'/'d'
- inconsistent spelling – same word is spelt in different ways on the same page
- wrong letter doubled – 'feel'/'fell'
- all letters present but not in the right order – 'poeple'; 'becuaes'; 'frist'

- incorrect word given with same letters – 'how' for 'who'; 'from' for 'form'
- difficulty with the short vowel sounds – 'cap'; 'pet'; 'kit'; 'hop'; 'cub'
- more difficulty with the long vowels – 'cape'; 'kite'; 'hope'; 'cube'
- further difficulty with vowel combinations – 'rain'; 'boat'; 'feet'; 'read'; 'loud'
- difficulty hearing the sounds of letters, the blends in a word – 'bl'; 'str'; 'gr'
- relying heavily on spelling phonetically to attempt unknown words – 'stashen' for 'station'; 'prite' for 'pretty'

**How you can help in the beginning**

1. Phonological awareness, learning the sounds to spell words

A dyslexic child will continue to have trouble with phonics (the sounds) of letters and their corresponding grapheme (letter symbol) beyond the age of seven or eight when most children will be getting to grips with them. Parents need to be aware that their dyslexic child needs much more time spent on the basic skills before really becoming confident in sound-symbol correspondence and word building.

Remember, and this is emphasized in almost every chapter – you are not a teacher at home, but you can certainly support your dyslexic child in his learning. If you feel it would be beneficial, then by all means follow a spelling programme such as Alpha to Omega or Synthetic Phonics. And it would be a very good idea to try out some computer software that assists in learning spelling, such as Wordshark and Hairy Letters. There are plenty of apps and games that you can check out for the early years. Knowledge of phonics is the key and enables the child to decode words (read) and encode words (spell).

## 2. Building a bank of sight words

Dyslexic children won't have a good visual skill for picturing words, even if they are great at picturing a 3-D model in their minds. The added drawback is that there are a lot of words that are not spelt phonetically and require visual memory.

Therefore it is a good idea to have a notebook of common words, including these illogical spellings – silent letters, exceptions to the rule, and so on. For example: 'believe', 'people', 'four', 'friend', 'could', 'because' ...

Check out lists of the most used words and the most commonly misspelt words and keep in a notebook. Particularly useful but hard-to-remember words can be put up around the home, or objects labelled in the kitchen, and so on.

## 3. Knowing the patterns of words and spelling rules

Spellings given at school can often be quite random and, as a dyslexic likes logic, this is not helpful for mastering the spelling of words. One way you can help is to encourage the grouping of word families and the learning of spelling rules, which could then be kept in a notebook and reviewed when necessary. For example: '-ight' words like 'bright'; '-dge' words like 'bridge'; '-tion' words like 'station'.

Make word families such as 'cat', 'mat', 'hat'; or 'light', 'might', 'sight', 'bright'; and encourage seeing patterns in words.

Play games – Boggle, Bananagrams, Pears, Word Slam, Word Dominoes, Syllable Snap ... whatever you can find.

## Coping with the Dreaded Weekly Spelling Tests

You may well be experiencing the challenges of the regular spelling test in school and trying hard to support your child, who is becoming more and more frustrated and disheartened by her lack of ability to spell.

The main issue for the dyslexic in this situation is not just the challenge of knowing the sequence of sounds, it is more crucially the weak working (short-term) memory. You will have been reviewing this week's spellings every day with your child only for most of them to be forgotten on the day of the test. Or, more usually, remembered almost perfectly for the test but not retained the next week when used in creative writing.

> 'I'd study and study, my brain was jumbling all over because there was a lot of stress and then I'd be guessing the words.'
>
> Sean, 13, remembering spelling tests

> 'I knew the spellings going to bed Thursday night and I'd wake up Friday morning and they'd be gone. When we'd get our results back, I'd be getting half of them wrong. I was hiding it from my parents, the embarrassment. I hid my tests in my bag. I'd lie about my results or just not bring it up.'
>
> Katie, 19, remembering spelling tests

A major problem with the weekly spelling test is that often a group of words is given to be taken home and learnt, but these words may not be used regularly or be meaningful for the child. Consequently, without regular use after the test the dyslexic child will completely forget the correct spellings.

The key is to be multi-sensory in their learning, where they can use more than one sense to reinforce a letter, a word, a sequence. This is a visual / auditory / kinaesthetic / tactile approach. So tap into your own creativity and that of your child's and see what multi-sensory ideas work. (More on this can be found in Chapter 8.)

· · · · · · · · · · · · · · · · · · · · · · · · · · · · · · · · · · · · · · ·

The 'look-say-cover' method is not enough.
Don't do that any more!

· · · · · · · · · · · · · · · · · · · · · · · · · · · · · · · · · · · · · · ·

> 'It just wouldn't go into my head as much as I'd try . . . I'd keep saying it over and over again.'
>
> Juliette, 17, remembering trying the traditional approach to learning spellings

## Some Fun Ideas to Help with Spellings

Here are some ideas which will be more useful, versatile and fun.

### Visual techniques

- Use colour highlighters for unusual letter patterns or the difficult part of the word.
- See the shape of the word – 'bridge'; 'flight'.
- Encourage seeing the word with a picture and in the mind's eye.
- Make a picture and story around the word.
- Write using plastic letters, foam letters or fridge magnet letters.
- Try texting the words as a phone message.
- Being aware of the vowels as early as possible is a good idea, so have the vowels in a word in a different colour.
- Use a whiteboard and lots of colours to practise spellings.

> 'Saying the letters out loud didn't help me . . . I'd need to see it. Coloured pens helped.'
>
> Caoimhe

### Auditory techniques

Don't just test the spellings on a car journey by asking for them out loud – this is stressful and does not help your child retain them.

- Sound out the word.
- Break up longer words – put a vertical line through syllable divisions. For example: 'in / vest / i / gate'.
- Clap or bang the beat of each syllable.
- Mnemonics (a device to help remember a sequence). For example, for the word 'because': 'big elephants can always upset smaller elephants'. Be careful with these, because for most dyslexic children with a bad short-term memory these little phrases are just something else for them to try to remember, and can be quite time-consuming. The sooner they can stop relying on this technique the better.
- Focus on word families with the same sound pattern.

'We sometimes do them in the car on the way to school . . . not fun!'

Anna, 9, on preparing for the weekly spelling test

### Kinaesthetic / tactile techniques

(the best channels for the dyslexic child – movement and touch)

- Trace the letters in a tray of sand, flour or on the table.
- Try writing the word with eyes closed.
- Make letters with Play-Doh, clay, pipe-cleaners.
- Try custard powder and water – a gooey texture and smells nice.
- Write the word with broad arm movements in the air – gross muscular movement.
- Use a mirror to see how vowel sounds and blends are formed in the movement of the mouth – see and feel the shape of the mouth while saying the word.

- Use beads, blocks, cotton reels to represent each sound, so then your child can physically place an object on the table to correspond to that sound. This is a good multi-sensory exercise – seeing, saying, moving and feeling.
- Often the short vowel sounds are difficult to discriminate – 'i' and 'e' in 'pit' and 'pet'. Try using kinaesthetic clues with little phrases, such as 'i' for 'itchy' and making a scratching mime.

'I like the pipe-cleaners; I can picture the letters all together after making them.'

Helena

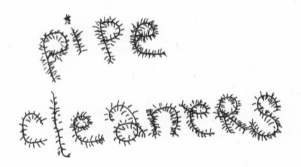

'I remember the feel of the sandbox and tracing on the table. I was such a moving-around person, up and down the hall and around the kitchen. All those interactive things really helped me, rather than sitting at the desk and staring over the paper, I couldn't do that at all.'

Katie, 19, remembering kinaesthetic learning of spellings

'I'd jump over a broomstick every time I'd get a word right. I'd pretend I was a horse as I like horse-riding. Every time you get a word right – kick a ball against the wall or whatever. It depends on what you like to do. Saying the word like a cheerleader was good, making the shape of the word and jumping up.'

Alannah's advice as a very kinaesthetic learner on how to keep motivated and make learning spellings fun

### The benefit of cursive writing (joined writing)

Cursive writing should be learnt and encouraged as soon as possible. Every time the pen is lifted from the page, there is more of a chance of an error when it is put down again. So it is best to help eliminate the possibility of errors by keeping the pen on the page with cursive handwriting. The flow from one letter to the next also has a kinaesthetic emphasis, always a bonus for the dyslexic. There are plenty of practice books for handwriting out there.

### Tackling the 'b'/'d' confusion

The difficulty distinguishing between 'b' and 'd' can continue right up to secondary school.

- 'bed' can be pencilled at the top of the page as a reminder
- use thumbs – left thumb up = 'b'; right thumb up = 'd'; and together they form 'bed'
- you can also check 'p' and 'q' with the thumbs down
- write in marker pen 'b' and 'd' on thumbs

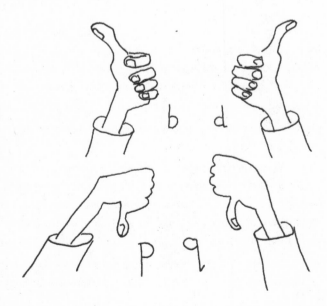

Here is some advice from parents who have already been through these years.

> 'Spellings were a nightmare! Try not to fight every day! If we did the spellings first it was better, before the writing, because they were so hard.'
>
> Yvonne

> 'Think creatively – tap into your own creativity as a dyslexic parent.'
>
> Danielle

However, you may find some of these wonderful creative ideas just frustrate your child even more. After all, this is learning spellings, not the most exciting activity.

> 'I wouldn't do well in any of them, the dread at the end of the week. Mum got these ideas – I used to trace the word with a light on the ceiling or picture the word with a giant 'A' in colour . . . I hated doing it!'
>
> Molly, remembering preparing for her spelling tests

## Creating a Personal Dictionary of Words

(See also Chapter 8 for more on a personal dictionary to help with poor working memory.)

You can use a simple little notebook or an address book if your child would prefer words alphabetically. A personal dictionary is useful for:

- new words a child wants to spell, meaningful words for creative writing or the latest topic in school
- words that your child frequently misspells

- word families, such as '-ight' words or words with the magic 'e': 'cape'; 'kite'
- words that have no logic, silent letters, and so on

It is important to make the strategy to remember the spelling of a word as memorable as possible.

- use colour, highlighters, draw the shape around the word: for example, noting the 'b', 'd' and 'g' in the word 'bridge'
- break up the word into its syllables, chunk the word – 'in / for / ma / tion'
- find words within words – 'to-get-her' = 'together'
- make pictures around the word: 'witch with a witch's hat' to remember the 't'
- put the word in a sentence
- have a definition if needed

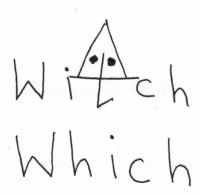

Never do more than four or five words in a week, and review these words for four weeks. By week three, your child should be just about able to write the words in a sentence without checking her strategy first.

The aim is for these more relevant words to pass into the long-term memory rather than being part of the mass of words remembered briefly for the Friday spelling test.

It is important these words are meaningful for your child and chosen by her. With regular reviewing and use of these words, your child will feel a sense of achievement and confidence in being able to spell.

## Multi-Sensory Ideas

Here is a guide to multi-sensory spelling, which you can combine with a personal dictionary.

---

**Multi-sensory strategies to help with spelling**

- know your learning strength – visual / auditory / kinaesthetic / tactile
- use your senses – see, hear, feel
- create your own strategy to remember a word
- chunk your word by sounds / syllables / visual clues
- make your word with plastic letters, pipe cleaners or Play-Doh
- trace your word on the desk or in sand or flour
- say your strategy
- see your word in your 'mind's eye'
- write your word in a sentence
- review for at least four weeks until your word is automatic for you
- use your word in your creative writing

---

---

Keep this six-step method as a handy reminder

First, create your visual strategy that will help you:

<u>Look</u>, <u>Say</u>, <u>Cover</u>, <u>Picture</u>, <u>Write</u>, <u>Check</u>

1. <u>Look</u> at the word and your strategy you've created
2. <u>Say</u> your strategy – the colours used, how you have broken it up
3. <u>Cover</u> it up and say your strategy again without looking
4. <u>Picture</u> the word in your mind's eye (the most important stage)
5. <u>Write</u> the word from memory, as it would be written in a sentence
6. <u>Check</u> you've got it right; if not – go through each stage once more

---

Sometimes, dyslexic individuals cannot picture a word in the mind's eye, which can make learning spellings a little more challenging, but this is where kinaesthetic–tactile learning can really be emphasized.

## Spelling in the Later Years

### Forget it!

Your focus on spelling is in the primary years. Just hope that some of those skills transfer to secondary school, because there won't be any time then to focus on spelling!

The challenge at secondary school, when spelling is no longer part of the learning, is that writing is more fluid and rushed, leading to more spelling errors in even the simplest of words. This brings obvious implications for self-esteem.

## Top Tips for Supporting a Dyslexic Teenager

- Don't focus too much on spelling, applaud content.

- Find out about assistive technology, see what you can get that will help with spelling ability, for example computer software with phonetic word prediction or phone apps.
- Be an advocate for your older child – communicate with school and make sure she isn't being marked down for spelling mistakes in her work. Remind them that she cannot help her poor spelling.

**CASE STUDY**

**NICOLA, REMEMBERING HER EXPERIENCES WITH SPELLING AT SECONDARY SCHOOL AND BEYOND**

'The main challenge was retaining the information that I just learnt. I got, and still get, mixed up sometimes with the simplest of words. In my essays in secondary school, they would always come back full of circles marking my spelling mistakes. I also found that if I hadn't written a word in a long time, I would forget how to spell it. I felt stupid and incompetent as I felt that I should have known at that stage what these spellings were.'

Comments on their work and in reports such as 'spelling poor', 'work on your spelling', 'careless spelling' are just frustrating and unhelpful, equal to a 'still can't see well' remark for a visually impaired student. So remind teachers that your child cannot help poor spellings when writing essays and under pressure. She finds it difficult to spot her mistakes.

'A lot of teachers don't know I'm dyslexic so they mark me down automatically. Once my English teacher knew I had the spelling and grammar waiver, my marks went right up really fast.'

Juliette, 17

- Fight for any reasonable accommodations in exams, such as a waiver from being marked on spelling and grammar in the language subjects (always a huge challenge for the dyslexic student).
- Encourage syllable division techniques – to help with the spelling of challenging words (in English and Science, for example), taking away the fear of big words as each short syllable is manageable.
- Your teenager may ask for help with proofreading essays. You may also find proofreading a challenge if you are dyslexic yourself, so rope in someone who is a good speller. Reading the text backwards to check for spelling is a good trick because then you are focusing on each word out of context rather than just quickly skimming through.
- A personal dictionary is useful at secondary school, too – collecting words your teenager frequently uses and misspells, or putting them on flashcards, Post-it notes or at the back of the subject's exercise book. But be prepared for this not to be kept up!

## Using technology

Fortunately, there's a great deal of technology available now that can really help:

- Hand-held spell checkers are available, or just use your phone's built-in checker.
- Spelling and grammar apps and computer software.
- Beware of the general spell checker on a laptop, as a word may be the correct spelling but not the one needed for the context. It won't distinguish between words that sound the same but have different spellings: 'there' / 'their'; 'meet' / 'meat'.... or common confusions when rushed, such as: 'who' / 'how', 'dose' / 'does'. Some students find they are not that useful and will actually hide errors.

'Make use of your phone – say the word and it comes up. When you can't find it in the dictionary because you don't have the right initial letter, the phone will give the correct spelling and the definition.'

Katie's idea

Ultimately, there is just so much you can do to help as a parent. Going into adulthood, a lot of these issues with spelling and punctuation will remain.

'What didn't help was people asking me why I can't spell that word, or why didn't I know when the letter 's' should be added or not, or why didn't I know when the apostrophe should be added or not. I still find this so hard to figure out! My spelling and grammar are not what they should be like for someone my age.'

Nicola, art critic

'I had the same challenge in secondary school, again in university, and continue to have the same challenge. This was frustrating at a young age but I have come to terms with the fact I will never win the Spelling Bee. Some techniques that helped were probably associating words and utilizing them more frequently. Now I can overcome this with spell check.'

Luke, engineer

## Home Tools to Support Spelling

### Phonics
Synthetic phonics
The Alpha to Omega programme
www.nessy.com – Hairy Letters app
www.wordshark.co.uk

**Games**

Bananagrams

Word dominoes

Boggle

**Personal dictionary**

Notebook or address book

**Multi-sensory tools**

Post-it notes, flashcards

Handwriting practice books

Coloured pens

Plastic or foam letters

Whiteboard, sand tray

Pipe-cleaners, Play-Doh, flour, custard powder

Beads, cotton reels

Small mirror

**Takeaways from Chapter 6**

- be understanding of the difficulties
- embrace multi-sensory strategies
- communicate with school to accommodate difficulties

## CHAPTER SEVEN

# Helping with Writing

'I really struggled with the syntax of a sentence. I'd have this great sentence in my head and I'm struggling to phrase it on the paper.'

Katie, 19

## Helping with Putting Pen to Paper

This chapter will look at aspects of writing for the dyslexic child at primary and secondary school, and how you can best help and support your child who is struggling, by providing:

- tools to tackle the mechanics of writing
- ways to enjoy being a creative writer
- solutions for note-taking
- support at exam time

Writing is often judged in terms of good spelling, and poor spelling can affect flow and creative expression for the dyslexic child. As with good reading and spelling skills, being able to write well is an emotive issue. Frustrations with writing and getting thoughts down on the page are a major part of having dyslexia.

There are three aspects in the skill of writing that are a challenge for the dyslexic child, and maybe for you, too:

1.  The mechanics of writing – knowing spellings, sentence structure, paragraphing, punctuation.
2.  The creative activity in writing – getting imaginative ideas and vocabulary down on the page. The ability to write interesting, expressive content.
3.  Being able to listen or read to take notes necessary for learning information, and with speed and accuracy.

## The Primary School Years

Learning to write is a challenge for all young children, and for the young dyslexic it is a skill that needs time, practice and reinforcement. There is so much for your child to master:

- the formation of the letters in the correct order for the word
- constructing a sentence so that it makes sense
- knowing when to use punctuation – full stops, commas, and so on
- using correct grammar
- knowing when to create a new paragraph
- being able to proofread and spot mistakes

And this is all before showing an ability to create stories and use expressive vocabulary! With the notoriously poor working memory and a difficulty in getting words down on the page, you can appreciate the frustrations, the tears, the anger, and the avoidance tactics that your child may use when it comes to writing. It is a mountain to climb for many.

'I thought I was writing a good story. I tried to avoid the bad spellings and use a different word and it just wouldn't work out for me.

People would want to see my story but I'd get embarrassed about my spelling, and they'd ask why had I got that simple spelling wrong.'

Aoife, 13, remembering writing stories at primary school

## Supporting the Mechanics of Writing

You cannot be a teacher at home, but you can give some help and encouragement towards your child becoming a competent writer. The whole process of writing a sentence is quite a challenge, needing practice and reinforcement. There is little you can do other than be supportive and understanding. Be there when it comes to written homework, and gently remind your child of sentence structure and punctuation.

A good idea is to maintain a bank of words commonly used as linking words in sentences, such as 'and', 'because', 'unless', 'although'. These can be put in a notebook or in the homework area.

You will also be helping your child to maintain her personal dictionary of words, and these would be words she wants to use for her free writing. With a growing confidence in the spelling of these words, her flow and expression in her writing will improve.

### The problem with handwriting

'I'd have to put my index finger between spaces, to make spaces between words, otherwise I'd write them all as one word.'

Alex, looking back on her early struggles in primary school

Children with dyslexia can struggle with writing by hand, but more so if they have dyspraxia or dysgraphia (see the Appendix for further information), which affect the fine motor skills in forming letters. Handwriting can be a real struggle as it takes up so much of the weak working memory, trying to remember how to form and join each letter, on top of how to spell the word.

There should be some practice in school, but there is no harm in also encouraging handwriting practice at home. There are plenty of practice books out there to learn cursive (joined) writing, as well as computer software like the program 'Handwriting without Tears'.

Handwriting practice probably won't be a very enjoyable exercise and focusing on letter formation could stultify any creative development when writing stories. Therefore, any opportunity to circumnavigate the actual physical writing and get straight to the story via an alternative route will be a bonus.

> 'I hated joined writing. I stopped doing it as soon as I could!'
>
> Juliette, 17

## Use of technology – typing skills

<u>Learning to touch-type is essential</u> for the dyslexic who struggles to write his thoughts by hand on the page. A lot of tears and clashes at home can be avoided, along with the opportunity of a confidence boost, if a keyboard is given as an option.

Touch-typing skills will offer more focus on other aspects of the writing process – sentence structure, grammar, paragraphing. The working memory that has been taken up with the formation of letters by hand can be freed up to concentrate on the other mechanics of writing.

> 'I'd much prefer it.'
>
> Luca, 10, on the option of typing stories

## Supporting the Creative Skills of Writing

When it comes to the creative side of writing, there are two types of dyslexic writers: those who cannot think of anything to put on to the page or develop, and those who are so full of creative ideas they want to write several chapters but don't know how to begin.

> 'I like making up stories. My problem is keeping it down – I want to write chapters.'
>
> Helena, 12

You may recognize your child as having elements of both types. Either way, they all need help with getting their thoughts down on paper in some kind of clear structure, as well as their desire to express themselves clearly and reflect their verbal intelligence.

> 'I like writing stories but the spelling sometimes is hard.'
>
> Anna, 9

### Valuing content above spelling
. . . . . . . . . . . . . . . . . . . . . . . . . . . . . . . . . . . . . .
Remember – just because they can't spell very well,
it doesn't mean they aren't good writers.
. . . . . . . . . . . . . . . . . . . . . . . . . . . . . . . . . . . .

Did the extraordinary and prolific authors Roald Dahl and Agatha Christie allow their lack of ability to spell well stop them from creating their imaginative characters and ingenious plots?

> 'I myself was always recognized as the "slow one" in the family. Writing and spelling were always terribly difficult for me.'[1]
>
> Agatha Christie

School reports in the Roald Dahl archives include teachers' comments:

> 'I have never met anybody who so persistently writes words meaning the exact opposite of what he obviously intended . . . quite incapable of marshalling his thoughts on paper.'[2]

> 'I loved his books when I was younger, and I thought you couldn't be a good writer with dyslexia. But it's the story that counts, so I just have to make the story and not worry about spelling.'
>
> Juliette, 17

A lot of children with dyslexia enjoy writing stories despite the challenges of spelling and the mechanics of writing. It is vital that you encourage this creativity and keep it separate from the boring mechanics. You will be making a huge difference to your child's self-belief, which may well be fragile because of the focus on spelling and punctuation at school.

You are not the teacher, you can praise your child for her amazing creativity and ideas, looking beyond the awkward spelling and lack of commas.

> 'When I read out a story I had written, my dad would be next to me and point out all my spellings – "You spelt that wrong . . . you spelt that wrong!" I'd get so annoyed about that. Don't look at the bad sides of it when they're showing you something, look at the creativity and content. Remember the spellings for later to help them.'
>
> Juliette's advice

## Helping with planning

'I could never start off a story by myself. I'd ask the teacher, "Can you just give me the first sentence?" Everyone else got better and I just stayed the same. I just wanted it done quickly.'

Abbie, 14, remembering writing at primary school

'I had it in my head all planned and that it would turn out really well but it never worked out like that for me.'

Aoife, 13, remembering writing at primary school

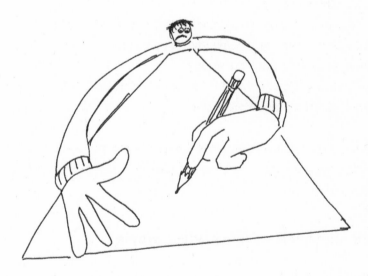

Children can find it difficult to start a story, especially when they have lots of ideas in their head but can't structure their creativity on the page. You could help by making sure your child gets used to planning his essays – a good habit to get into as early as possible. There are many students who never plan their essays right through their school career, and this is always reflected in their output. The sooner your child knows the advantages of planning all essays and pieces of work, the better for his future academic success. Once the planning is second nature for him, then your work is done in this area. A variety of approaches might help:

- Discuss the story ideas with your child – this is the most enjoyable part usually, and very helpful for your child to generate ideas and formulate a plan.
- Brainstorm ideas with what is sometimes called a 'spider-gram' – a central circle with lots of ideas coming off it. This is very effective for those dyslexic children who find it hard to come up with ideas, as well as those who need all their ideas to be reined in.
- If a more linear list is preferred, the '5Ws, 1H' prompter is very good to focus attention and bring logical content to a story – 'what, where, when, who, why, how' questions.
- Have a collection of objects, such as a key, a shell, a piece of jewellery, which can then inspire a story.

With these approaches, there is a danger of entering teacher territory, so make sure you just instil the importance of planning as part of the skill of writing, and then leave them to it.

### Finding alternative ways to produce writing

'I'd be flying along, I'd feel like my brain is going a hundred times faster than my hand and I'd have all my ideas.'

Katie, 19, remembering writing essays

Part of the tears and frustration for the dyslexic child with an essay assignment is that feeling of being unable to get all those good ideas from the creative mind down on paper. How discouraging to know that all these fabulous words and ideas are in the brain but can never get transferred to the written word. And however hard they try, the dyslexic child is exhausted after his written attempt, and then judged by the teacher as not having made enough effort.

The best thing you can do in this situation is find an alternative way for your child to get his great stories out there, and show to the teacher and to himself that, yes, he has ability and could go on to be very good at English, given the chance.

Alternatives are needed to prevent this loss of flow and creativity through the laborious physical act of writing. Here are some options:

- Dictation – your child could dictate his story to you and you could act as a scribe, writing down his story for him or typing it
- Record him telling his story and transcribe the result
- Get him into touch-typing as soon as possible, taking away the physical formation of letters, and with spell checker he will focus more on his creativity, though giving him complete freedom to tell his story out loud is the best option
- Use assistive technology such as voice-activated software, which will write what is spoken, for example Dragon Naturally Speaking
- Make sure you have lots of different-coloured eraser pens for your child who hates to make mistakes – she will enjoy writing far more if she can correct mistakes without having crossed-out words or making a mess on the page

---

**CASE STUDY**

**LUCA**

Luca will spend a long time agonizing over a sentence when he has to write by hand, but he has found a love of writing poems since being able to dictate what is coming to his very creative and intelligent mind. Here is one of his poems, inspired by the colour red.

Red

Autumn harvest has failed and the villagers are falling

Soldiers fight, the red sun glowing behind them

Blood squirting out of dead squires

The King's axe covered with anger

The foe is being lit up with flames

Victory is ours, the red flags are flying, happiness is rising

Reproduced by kind permission of Luca Kavanagh, 10

---

**Liaising with the class teacher**

One of the most significant issues for any dyslexic individual is that written work does not reflect your verbal intelligence. This is shown very clearly in Luca's poem. Your child may be having very negative experiences when it comes to writing in school. Teachers may not realize your child's language ability and neither may your child realize his ability.

Communicate with the school and ask for alternative ways for your child to produce work, such as orally or through the use of computers. The school, the child and his peers may be pleasantly surprised by the outcome. If alternative formats aren't forthcoming, then request that your child writes less than his peers, but without 'dumbing down' his work.

## Helping with the Challenges of Note-Taking

'I'd have to write one letter and look back and then up ... I'd be writing each letter and taking so much longer.'

Aoife, remembering taking notes in primary school

'I couldn't write the sentence in the time given, I just wouldn't get to the answer.'

Sarah, remembering taking notes in primary school

People with dyslexia have a poor working memory, a poor ability to retain the image of a word or a spelling. So being able to remember what they see on the board and transfer that to their notes is quite a challenge.

It takes a while for the dyslexic child to copy down each letter, each word, and invariably the meaning and comprehension of the content is lost at the same time. They quickly realize from primary school onwards that they don't have the skills in note-taking that their peers seem to take for granted.

### Ways you can help

All you can do is communicate with your child's teacher if it is becoming an issue and she is missing out on some of the learning in class. See if it is possible to have notes transferred more often to diagrams, mind-maps and pictures, or to receive a hand-out of the important information. Ready-made notes supplied by the overworked teacher would be ideal but not always possible.

Make sure your child isn't being kept behind in class to finish copying from the board when the rest of the class is outside for playtime. That is cruel and unfair; your child cannot help her short-term memory issue and her need for more time to take down sentences in her own hand.

There are always alternative ways to take notes – computers, word processors and spell checkers are becoming more and more common and an accepted part of the classroom. Encourage fluency on the keyboard, find touch-typing programmes to practise at home and build a proficiency that will give your child the confidence to write as she desires.

## Writing in Secondary School and the Teenage Years

'In secondary school, I found that writing essays, especially in History, Geography and English, were the most difficult. I couldn't write as quickly as anyone else, I couldn't write as much as anyone else and my writing wasn't as extensive as the rest of the class.'

Nicola, art critic

Transition to secondary school is a huge leap for all children for many reasons, but for a dyslexic child the new challenges in reading and writing can be particularly daunting. Imposing tasks include the expectation put on first-year students to produce well-developed written answers and long essays, as well as competent notes for their studies.

Unfortunately, the stresses and difficulties with writing at primary school just increase once your child is in secondary school. The pressure to write well, accurately and fast in class and in exams becomes a major obstacle for the intelligent and quite probably verbally articulate dyslexic student.

The young dyslexic student is overwhelmed by it all, and although he feels he is working hard and is exhausted by the concentration and effort needed to write, he is perplexed to find teachers' comments on his work admonishing him for not developing his answers and, of course, being careless with spelling and punctuation.

No wonder a young student may feel like giving up, avoiding homework altogether, or feel he just isn't any good at school.

So how can you help your older child, now dealing with the demands of secondary school and the new curriculum?

First, you need to have some understanding of what your child is going through, so you can give empathy and encouragement, but also communicate with the school and educate teachers about his difficulties, such as why the written work he is producing is not reflecting his ability.

## Particular challenges for the older child and teenager

- plenty of thoughts and ideas but struggles to express these clearly and fluently on the page
- writing block when sitting down to write – just can't start
- lots of ideas on the page but no proper structure or continuity
- writing exacerbated by poor handwriting that is slow and laborious
- difficulty keeping up with listening and taking notes in class
- can't take down all the notes from the board before they are erased
- can't process answers fast enough in an exam situation
- written work doesn't reflect verbal intelligence
- rewriting sentences to avoid more interesting words unable to spell – a dumbing-down of oneself
- the whole idea of having to write is stressful, instilling panic or revulsion
- exhausted by it all

Some dyslexic teenagers explain their difficulties with writing:

> 'I wasn't good at phrasing things economically, I'd write around the point and not to the point.'
>
> Molly, 19

> 'I know what I'm saying in my head, I just don't know how to put it into words. It's so frustrating.'
>
> Abbie, 14

> 'I'm looking ahead; I can't catch up with my own brain when I'm writing, so I miss out words.'
>
> Sean, 13

> 'You'd go into an exam and you'd know it and you'd be writing it down and then, "Oh no . . . what comes after that?" And then you'd just have passed that sentence and your brain would be trying to track it back and it's gone from your mind then.'
>
> Katie, 19

## Helping with Writing Challenges

### Planning and structuring skills

Stay away! You can make suggestions, but as we explore in Chapter 9, you will only add to their stresses and frustrations if you get too involved in the writing process at this stage of their school career. Trust that the school is teaching the skills needed to plan and answer questions. Just encourage planning as part of the writing process, and explain that it will make life easier for them in the long run. It is, in fact, the most important stage when a student is feeling overwhelmed by a writing task. They need to feel in control and confident they can do it.

'It is just harder to get my ideas down on the page. I used to just jump straight in and not know where I was going. But now I can plan it and know where I'm going with it.'

Emily, 18

- Supply a whiteboard, Post-it notes, coloured pens and eraser pens – equipment conducive to brainstorming ideas and trial and error.
- Be available to listen to your older child explain his ideas for an essay. Being able to talk through his ideas to someone else will help him clarify for himself the structure of his answer.
- Get outside help – a professional who can help brainstorm and organize essay structures, thus avoiding any teenage clashes with you.
- Technology is always there – check out computer software and encourage its use to help with planning, such as www.inspiration.com.

## Proofreading

A dyslexic will often assume he is seeing on the page what he had in his mind to put on the page. However, there will be words missing and errors in punctuation that he will probably not notice.

- offer to read the finished piece out loud for him
- you may also find proofreading a challenge with your own dyslexia, so enlist the help of someone else to read the piece out loud
- text-to-speech software can also assist greatly with proofreading any pieces of work

## Note-taking

'I feel like I'm not fast enough taking notes. I don't have them all, I have bits of different notes. When I read over it, it doesn't make sense, it's loads of bits just put together.'

Aoibhinn, 14

The greatest demand on a dyslexic student's writing skills comes with note-taking in secondary school. Non-dyslexics take it for granted that they can hold a phrase or sentence in their minds and write it down, as well as absorb the sense of what they are writing. They can also listen to someone and pick out the key words to make their own notes.

This is a very challenging skill for most dyslexics. Their bad short-term memory prohibits full retention of what the person has said, added to the need to concentrate on the mechanics of spelling and make sure notes are legible and comprehensible. Often their notes aren't of any value when it comes to studies later on, as so much has been missed and confused, and the context of that lesson has long gone from the memory.

It is a wonder that dyslexic students are so capable of achieving so much in their school careers. They show a determination and strength of character that others may not realize. Dyslexic students on average have to work four times harder than their peers to achieve equivalent results.

Here are some practical ways you can help with note-taking:

- Liaise with the teachers at the parent–teacher meetings and request hand-outs of important notes.
- Find good revision books in subjects – look for clear bullet points, plenty of spacing, colour and diagrams (dyslexia-friendly).
- Offer different-coloured A4 pads of paper – dyslexic students are more likely to prefer making notes on a colour other than white. This does not mean that all dyslexics prefer yellow paper and blue ink. All sorts of colours appeal.
- Supply plenty of highlighter pens and eraser pens to support whatever way your teenager prefers to take notes.
- If your teen is more of a listening learner than a visual learner, then

ask permission to record lessons that can be played back later to make notes.

- They may prefer to listen to information without the distraction of taking notes, and can absorb much more detail this way.

> 'I don't take notes in class, I just listen . . . I can't take notes in class, or I'll miss something.'
>
> Caoimhe, 14

- Make use of technology – typing notes can be very beneficial, besides the fact that the student's notes are clearer to read, there are fewer spelling errors and more opportunity to create notes visually. The working memory can be freed up from the act of writing by hand to make room for creative processes, such as mind-mapping. Speech-to-text software is also great as it allows the student to dictate notes and essays, and the program is able to translate his speech into printed text.

> 'You are trying to concentrate on your spelling and what you're trying to say and form a sentence that makes sense, it's a lot to focus on. Typing is a muscle memory; you don't have to concentrate on your writing. You can focus on what you are actually saying and not how you're writing it down.'
>
> Leah, 18

There cannot be a right or wrong way to take in information and process it. The right way is whatever suits your child, and you can only offer alternatives and encourage him to have confidence in how he prefers to learn.

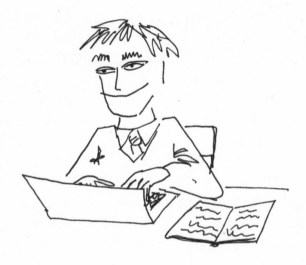

## Being an Advocate and Ensuring Equal Opportunity in Exams

(See Chapter 11 for more on being an advocate.)

You want your teenager to have as much chance as his peers to show what he is capable of in his school exams. Therefore, you must push for any reasonable accommodations open to him. Having a spelling and grammar waiver, a scribe or a laptop can be extremely liberating for the dyslexic student who struggles to get his thoughts on paper in the time given, and consequently questions his own capabilities. You don't want him to give up on his talents before he realizes his potential. Options may include:

- extra time – for example, an extra ten minutes per hour of an exam
- access to a laptop for all written assignments and exams
- use of a scribe to write for the student who dictates his answers
- use of computer software to record answers, such as speech-to-text

- own room given for the exams to reduce distractions and anxiety
- breaks given to allow physical movement or to deal with anxiety

NB – it must be noted here that you may find most of these options are only open to students who have other specific difficulties, such as dyspraxia or dysgraphia. Having dyslexia alone may not allow a student to have access to these accommodations, which can be extremely frustrating for both student and parent.

Once the dyslexic has been liberated from the constraints of transferring what's in his brain to the written word, the results can be surprising for the teachers, for you the parent and, most significantly, for the child. He now realizes that he isn't slow or stupid compared to his siblings and peers. He can achieve just as well or better than them. Many individuals with dyslexia have the potential to become highly skilled writers and achievers, given the opportunity.

If your child is resistant to using these accommodations, and doesn't want to be seen as 'different', it is important to let him know these accommodations are positive and there for him to have the same opportunities as his classmates. Remember – it is not cheating, it is not an unfair advantage and, yes, it will probably make a difference to his marks and show what he is capable of (teachers may need to be told this, too).

...........................................

Appropriate accommodations are essential to unlock potential for a dyslexic student. They remove the barriers that prevent dyslexic individuals from expressing what they know.

...........................................

'For me, what really helped was the fact I had a spelling and grammar waiver all through secondary school . . . this allowed me to write words I would not dare try and spell before.'

Luke, engineer

'The scribe really helped. You don't have to worry about spelling or forgetting words. There is nothing holding you back from saying complicated words. It's the scribe's job to spell it, not yours!'

Sarah, 15

See Chapter 10 and Chapter 11 for more on exam support and self-confidence.

## Home Tools to Support Writing Skills

### Handwriting practice books

### Stationery
notebooks, Post-it notes
coloured A4 pads
whiteboard
coloured pens and highlighters
eraser pens

### Revision books in school subjects

### Graphic organizers for planning

### Assistive technology
touch-typing skills – lots of free sites and apps
speech-to-text software (e.g. Dragon Naturally Speaking)
planning software (e.g. www.inspiration.com)

## Takeaways from Chapter 7

- value content over spelling
- liaise with school for a range of support strategies
- encourage the skills of planning and structuring
- find alternative ways to create the written word

## CHAPTER EIGHT

# Working Memory – The Challenges of Forgetfulness

'My mind slips away from focus and I can't remember one certain part.'

Sean, 13

## Strategies and Techniques to Tackle a Poor Memory

This chapter will provide various strategies and techniques to help your child's poor working memory. It looks at the specific challenges relating to primary and later school years by providing:

- fun ways to remember spellings
- multi-sensory ideas for rote learning
- tools for getting the dyslexic child organized at secondary school
- ideas to support home study

Working memory, also known as short-term memory, can be defined as a mental workspace that stores and uses information for a short period of time. It is constantly active as we negotiate our often busy and challenging daily lives at work and at home.

There is a widespread notion that dyslexia is purely a difficulty with reading and spelling, but as emphasized in Chapters 1 and 2, the greatest challenge and frustration for children with dyslexia is their poor working memory.

> 'My memory frustrates me, I'm fine with reading and spelling, it doesn't bother me! But I just can't get the answer out of my head.'
>
> Emma, 17

Is your child being labelled as having poor concentration and easily distracted? Is your child being punished for being careless in school, forgetting textbooks and homework? Are you constantly reminding the dyslexics in your family to organize themselves, remember books, equipment and appointments?

You will see that in reality the greatest challenge associated with dyslexia is this forgetfulness. You may see it in yourself if you are also dyslexic. So this chapter will be invaluable for making home life a little easier.

## CASE STUDY

### YVONNE, PARENT, REFLECTING ON HER EXPERIENCES OF THREE SONS WITH DYSLEXIA

'I have three children and they all have dyslexia and show different traits, but disorganization is a trait across all of them. For me, the disorganization and the memory would be a huge issue. Losing stuff all the time is all to do with Aaron's dyslexia. Shane was always getting notes for forgetting things. So you just write it in their journal: "I appreciate he's getting all these notes for forgetting pencils and so

> on but, as you know, this is a difficulty with him, and if there could be a little leeway . . ."
>
> 'Parents can educate teachers about the short-term memory problems. Part of his dyslexia is that he forgets everything, but he does try. The spellings were the most stressful and I don't think they ever learnt anything off ever, it just didn't happen.'

There can be no magic wand or cure for a poor working memory, but at least we can work on the dyslexic strengths with various strategies and techniques to compensate for any weaknesses. And encouragingly, a past World Memory Champion, crowned a record eight times, is the dyslexic Dominic O'Brien. So there is hope!

## The Challenges of a Poor Memory – the Early Years

The primary years can be a very challenging and exposing time for the dyslexic child who is struggling with a weak working memory. Sadly, these symptoms of dyslexia may go unnoticed for a long time. These traits are then labelled as laziness, carelessness, lacking concentration or assumed to be a sign of low ability. The reality is that the child in primary school is struggling to remember everything – multiplication tables, spellings for the test on Friday, what the teacher just told the class to do and what homework needs to be done.

> 'I'm forgetting what I'm reading half the time.'
>
> Aoife

### How poor working memory manifests in the primary school years

You may notice some or all of the following in your dyslexic child during their early years at school:

- difficulty learning songs, learning months of the year and birthdays
- difficulty following routines and sets of instructions
- having to work so hard to learn spellings for tests, to then forget them completely afterwards
- almost impossible to learn the multiplication tables by rote; they just don't make sense
- not being able to remember what they did in school that day
- it seems conventional learning techniques just don't work
- teachers say they are careless, not concentrating and need to put more effort in
- exhausted after a day in school putting so much effort into trying to remember everything

'When my son was in senior infants, he had a problem remembering colours . . . when shown the colour green he would say it's the colour of grass. When reading his school book, he would recognize a word on one page but have completely forgotten it on the next page.'

Therese, parent

'Days of the week? Forget about it! Months of the year? Don't know! Simple rhymes I wouldn't have got. It didn't make sense, didn't compute.'

Mike, reflecting on his early primary school years

'Writing it out three times doesn't work.'

Abbie

'Anybody new I'd have to say their name at least five times just to get it into my brain for an hour, then I would have to say it another five times. Homework was the worst time of day, and I'd have no time to play.'

Roan, 11, reflecting on early primary school years

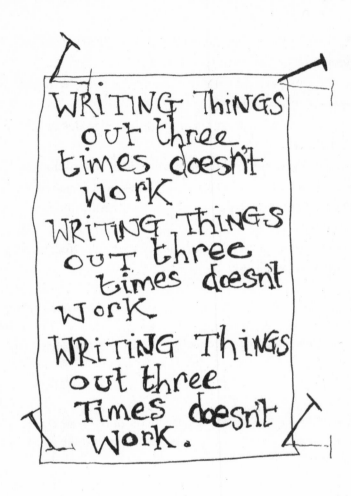

The primary years can be the toughest time if there is a lack of understanding of this significant issue for children with dyslexia. Awareness and intervention as early as possible is the key, and this is where you step in with one of your most important roles.

### Be an advocate for your child

(See Chapter 11 for more on this.) Tell the school about the working-memory difficulties that are aspects of your child's dyslexia. You can help the school and class teacher to understand that dyslexia is the reason for a lot of the difficulties your child is experiencing. (If dyslexia has not been spotted yet then these common symptoms need to be picked up on and worked with as soon as possible.) You want to make sure your child has a positive experience of school, so the earlier you know what it is and how you can help, the better.

. . . . . . . . . . . . . . . . . . . . . . . . . . . . . . . . . . . . . . . .

Don't despair, and don't feel bad.
You're here now, and there are practical things that you can do to help.

. . . . . . . . . . . . . . . . . . . . . . . . . . . . . . . . . . . . .

The working-memory weakness is where parents can really make a difference in terms of the practical help you can give.

> 'Parents need to tell teachers about organizing and memory difficulties. It put everything into perspective for her (the teacher).'
>
> Yvonne, parent

## All children learn differently

What is your child good at learning and remembering? There will be some things the dyslexic child can be relied upon to remember, such as song lyrics, directions to somewhere, dance moves, films and images. And she will have particular abilities, such as mechanical, artistic, musical, storytelling, dramatic arts, sports and so on.

Help your child to see what she is good at and how she can use her abilities to support her memory. By being multi-sensory, a child can use all her senses to aid her learning and remembering in the more challenging areas.

'What was good was learning how I learn as early as possible – learning what works for you to learn, what you're good at learning, what you're good at doing.'

Roan

Let's look at two key areas that cause a lot of stress and tears for both parent and child: (i) learning the weekly spellings; and (ii) learning the times tables.

## Learning Weekly Spellings

You may well experience the tears and frustrations as you try to help your dyslexic child with the list of words for the Friday spelling test. You have been reviewing and testing these words for three days leading up to the test. Maybe you have tried pictures, fridge magnets and reciting the spellings in the car on the way to school. Unfortunately, however hard you work on these words, they will be forgotten right after the test, unless these words are being used regularly and meaningfully.

'Spellings she would learn every day for her weekly spelling test would be forgotten by Friday morning, so basically she gave up.'

Colleen, parent, remembering her daughter's experience

'In twenty minutes you teach them ten spellings that they'll forget tomorrow – what is the point? It's just tears and frustrations, and not a good time spent together.'

Danielle, parent

### Making spellings more meaningful – a personal dictionary
(See more on this in Chapter 6.)
Encourage your child at primary level to maintain a notebook of words she wants to be able to spell for her day-to-day writing and creative

stories. This will make the arduous process of learning the spelling of words have more meaning and purpose. This personal dictionary will have words she wants to spell with her own strategies to help trigger her memory.

Let's look at multi-sensory ideas that could aid the learning of the correct spelling of words in the personal dictionary, as well as how you can help to create more efficient ways to learn those dreaded Friday spellings.

## Auditory (listening) learning

- sound out the word
- break down longer words to their syllables, clap or bang the beat of each syllable (a syllable is the beat in a word; it must include a vowel or 'y' acting as a vowel (e.g. the word 'syllable' has three syllables)
- learn word families with the same sound pattern – 'goat', 'coat', 'coal', 'foal'
- use cotton reels or other similar objects to represent each sound of a word and arrange into their blends, for example 'smash' would be the cotton reels arranged thus – ## # ## = sm a sh
- say out loud the personal strategy for the spelling of the word from the personal dictionary

## Visual learning

- encourage seeing the word in 'the mind's eye'
- use colour highlighters to highlight the difficult parts of the word
- make a picture to create a story around the word
- use plastic letters / foam letters to make the word
- see words within words. For example: 'cap / a / city'
- break up the word into sections: 'beau – ti – ful'
- see the shape of the word – 'enjoy'

'Different colours help, seeing the words in different colours – I can picture them better.'

Helena

'The "e" would be an elephant and we'd make a story with all of that. Every word would have a whole story to it. That was fun, making pictures.'

Roan

## Kinaesthetic / tactile (doing, making, touching) learning

This is the most important learning channel for the dyslexic child and, fortunately, it is the most fun to practise for the child struggling with remembering spellings.

- have a sand tray – a large container filled with sand (from the beach or sold at a large toyshop or DIY outlet) to write the word in; this is a particularly popular technique
- write the word with eyes closed
- trace the word on the desk or table
- write with broad arm movements in the air
- make the word with pipe-cleaners, clay or Play-Doh – another very popular and beneficial technique

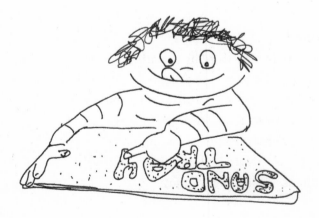

····················································

Remember – writing the word out three, five or twenty times does not work.

····················································

'Be patient, especially with spellings, which can be written out with colours or put on a board or outlined in sand.'

Lisa, parent of two young girls with dyslexia

'By the end of it we would have made up a story, drawn some pictures, done an animation and learnt the spellings.'

Danielle, parent

## Learning Times Tables

Some children with dyslexia have no problem with learning their multiplication tables. Many dyslexic children are gifted in the area of numbers and mathematics. However, a majority of these children struggle with the rote learning of their tables, which they see as illogical and impossible to master. Ultimately, they will be able to rely on technology at secondary school, but in the meantime at primary level they will experience the excruciating embarrassment and frustration of not knowing their tables in a class test.

### Some multi-sensory ideas to help with rote learning

Auditory (listening and speaking) strategies:
- recite the times tables out loud, or whatever needs to be learnt in a sequence
- listen to an audio recording
- create a song, use the tune of a nursery rhyme

Visual strategies:

- have Post-it notes around the room of the particular multiplication table being learnt, possibly different times tables per room, if you have the space
- test the times tables on a whiteboard
- see patterns in the times tables – the nines have an interesting pattern
- use colour to emphasize the difficult parts, the patterns

Kinaesthetic / tactile (doing, making, touching) strategies:

- write the times tables on a whiteboard or in a sand tray
- walk around, reciting the tables out loud
- walk to each Post-it note in the study space, recite out loud, and then recite without looking, by picturing each multiplication in its place in the room
- always fidget and walk around to help concentration

'I'm able to learn differently, in more fun ways.'

Daniel

---

## Helping Memory in the Early Years

- a notebook for a personal dictionary
- a tray of sand
- Play-Doh, clay
- pipe cleaners
- cotton reels
- plastic / foam letters
- Post-it notes
- colour highlighter pens
- a whiteboard
- audio recording equipment and software

## Secondary School Years

Poor working memory becomes the greatest frustration at secondary school, and a cause of much of the stress and disappointment in school work and exams for the dyslexic student.

'My memory card is full, my brain is full of the stuff that other people let go, and I can't keep hold of the school-related books.'

Cian, 17

'I could study Biology and forget it two hours later, and I've studied it for about two hours trying to figure it out, and it's gone.'

Julie, 17

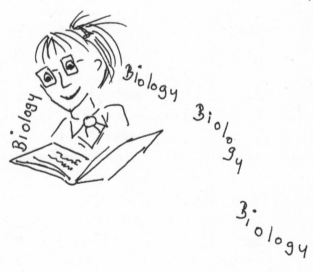

## Transition from Primary to Secondary School

The poor working memory is stretched to its limit in this transition. Suddenly, the dyslexic child is bombarded by new subjects, a timetable of different classrooms, textbooks, exercise books, homework journals, sports equipment, and so on. Before long, she is getting notes home for forgetting homework, her PE kit, her science textbook.

'The different rooms and teachers and names – organization is going to go out the window!'

Roan's concerns about transition to secondary school

'He was completely and utterly overwhelmed.'

Yvonne, parent, reflecting on her son's transition to secondary school

Learning new topics and studying for weekly tests become a huge challenge, often resulting in exhaustion, forgetting what has been learnt and, worst of all, going blank in the test that the dyslexic student spent hours trying to prepare for.

'In a test, you can't remember the answers and afterwards everyone says it was easy, but you couldn't remember half of it.'

Alannah, 13

The demand for further rote learning does not help matters. Now, rather than learning multiplication tables, your older child must learn scientific definitions, Shakespeare quotes, mathematical equations. And it is very apparent that the conventional learning techniques are not working.

With the added time pressure, the challenge of time management (which is never a dyslexic strength), and the workload building up, the dyslexic student has a working-memory overload and becomes more forgetful, exhausted and stressed. Consequently, secondary school can be an anxious, stressful experience, particularly in the early stages when a new student is trying to settle in.

'I sometimes cry with frustration.'

Sean

## How You Can Help with Organization and Study Time

There are two areas where parents can make a difference, and alleviate some of this anxiety and stress: (i) organization; and (ii) homework and exam study.

### Getting the dyslexic child organized at secondary school

'A huge problem at home – a lot of nagging! You'd know their timetable and double check they have gym gear in the bag as they go out the door. But you have to give them responsibility to do it for themselves as well.'

Yvonne, parent of three dyslexic sons

You are not policing your child's organization but you can make a lot of difference to his forgetfulness, disorder and stress. It is a careful balance of being supportive but also encouraging self-reliance.

- Be aware of the challenges transferring to secondary school and make allowances for poor memory at times – he can't help it.
- Make sure he has a routine for clearing out his school bag daily and packing it at night for the following day; this will reduce the chance of being punished by teachers for forgetting books.
- Have the school timetable in a prominent position; for example, in the kitchen, where other family members can remind him when sports equipment, musical instruments and so on need to be brought into school.
- Use colour – there are some great colourful stickers that can be used to colour-code textbooks, exercise books and hardbacks in each subject, so they can be easily found and sorted into the school bag. Also coloured sticky reminders are handy for the homework journal.

- A homemade timetable with lists of what books are needed for each section of the day can be useful for the forgetful student, and placed inside his school locker for double-checking.
- If forgetting books is the biggest issue for your dyslexic child, then consider having two sets of textbooks – one for home and one for school.

'I put up a whiteboard in her bedroom, so that the important stuff to be remembered could be written up there in big writing.'

Niamh, parent of a teenage dyslexic

'I want to keep stuff colour-coded because that's much easier than looking at names every single time.'

Roan

'Sticky notes by my bed help me to remember to put something in my bag.'

Juliette

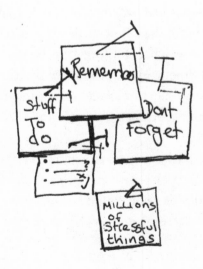

## Dealing with a poor memory at homework and study time

(See Chapter 9 and Chapter 10 for more on this.)

<u>Create a calm space for homework and study</u>

This can be a flashpoint at home between parent and child, and you may get frustrated with your dyslexic teen who has left essential books at school, hasn't written the homework down and seems unable to focus on any study.

- Make allowances for tiredness and forgetfulness – she can't help it, she has to work four times harder than her peers to stay afloat.
- Make sure she has a quiet study space, uncluttered and free from distractions.
- Offer files and folders and shelving so she can sort her subject notes and loose bits of paper.

'Basically trying to keep my daughter organized – a whiteboard in her bedroom with the class timetable, notes where PE clothes or cooking ingredients are needed for Home Economics. The timetable reviewed nightly to see what is required for the next day. And trying to keep the study area clear of clutter! Using different-coloured plastic envelope-type folders for each subject to hold, for example, the English book, poetry book, copy book and so on, so that for each subject in secondary school only one folder has to be taken from the locker at break time.'

Colleen, listing what she and her teenage daughter have found beneficial

<u>Support for your dyslexic teen studying for tests</u>

'You revise loads before and you know it all before the exam, and then once you hit the chair in the exam your mind goes blank.'

Luca, 14

The best thing you can do is encourage your dyslexic child to explore multi-sensory strategies for learning, as shown at primary level earlier in this chapter. Knowing how to learn and what suits his right-brained strengths is vital for the dyslexic student at secondary school.

Encourage your dyslexic child to tap into what he is good at remembering in everyday life, and to use his creativity to gain confidence in new multi-sensory ways of studying. Whether he is a first-year just starting out or soon to move on from secondary school, it is never too late to experiment and change ways to study.

> 'Parents need to see when something isn't working and is getting stressful – the route we're going down is clearly not working. The child is getting tired and frustrated and not really learning what they're supposed to be learning so, instead of going continuously down this track, let's try something else, like mind-maps, graphs or, instead of mind-maps, let's try a more linear-bullet-points, semi-structured notes system.'
>
> Mike, a graduate with dyslexia, advising parents on ways to help

## Practical help and the need to make allowances

### Auditory learning

- Encourage her to discuss and explain a difficult topic with you, such as photosynthesis in Biology. By having to explain the topic in her own words to someone else, she is better able to consolidate her own understanding of that topic for herself. Don't be a teacher – don't quiz her, just listen!

> 'It helps when I can explain the work I have done.'
>
> Katie, 16

'My mum goes over with me what we've been learning in Science and English.'

Sean, 13

- Help to create mnemonics to learn a sequence (often very difficult for a dyslexic student), such as the one we learnt at primary school for the colours of the rainbow – 'Richard Of York Gave Battle In Vain'.
- Allow her to play music in the background or through headphones. This is controversial, of course, but contrary to what you may think, music can aid concentration and block out other distractions around the dyslexic learner. Obviously some music will be more conducive, such as light classical. Mike makes this point overleaf.

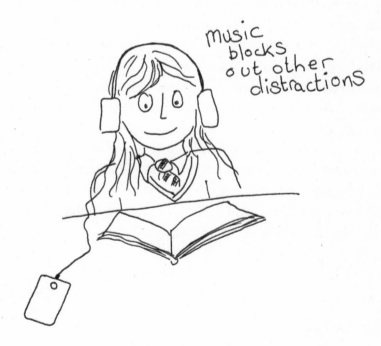

'Music blocks out everybody else in the house.'

Josh, 16

'I get more distracted by the lack of noise. You don't like the sound of nothing, especially if you're an audio learner. Music can cut out other sounds in the house – siblings, pets, etc. Not R&B or heavy metal or hip hop, obviously, something gentler, but something you like.'

Mike's advice as an auditory learner

### Visual learning

- Allow her to put Post-it note reminders and posters of study mind-maps on the walls in her study space, and even around the home, a different subject per room!
- Consider having different-coloured paper for each subject, and coloured A4 pads; for example, pale shades of blue, purple, yellow and green. Different colours suit different students.
- Give her an A3-size whiteboard for her to revise and test herself.
- Help her to find useful YouTube videos in challenging topics, such as History, Science and Geography.
- Encourage her to see in her 'mind's eye' if she has a good visual memory. Some dyslexic individuals don't picture things at all and are more auditory learners.
- Encourage mind-mapping if she is good at remembering where she saw something on a page. However, mind-mapping doesn't work for every dyslexic and can confuse a topic. Mind-maps are also time-consuming but, if a student perseveres, she may find they are a good way to recall information in the long term.

'Mind-maps help me to make connections.'

Cian, 17

'I like writing quotes out on flashcards in different ways.'

Juliette, 17

'It helps to draw it, like the volcano in Geography. I can remember what it looks like and the labels.'

Alannah, 13

## Kinaesthetic / tactile learning

- Don't be surprised to find him walking up and down and around the place reciting definitions and quotes out loud – encourage that.
- Supply plenty of flashcards of various colours and sizes that can be used to review key notes frequently.
- Possibly liaise with the school for your child to be an official 'fidgeter', not reprimanded but encouraged to play around with Blu Tack, elastic bands, pens or whatever works for him in class – this can aid concentration.

'I think better when I'm walking around.'

Ben, 16

'The teacher gives me Blu Tack for under the table in class, and there's always spare Blu Tack for me at home.'

Aoibhinn, 14

The main thing is to encourage and support any less conventional ways of studying. Let your dyslexic child tap into her creative strengths and simply help her along the way if needed.

'Once I found a way to study, and it was actually staying in my head, I got so excited.'

Nina, 17

## Home Tools to Aid Memory and Organization in Secondary School

- files and folders for school subjects
- two sets of textbooks for home and school
- stickers of varied colour and shape
- flashcards
- coloured paper and A4 pads
- highlighter pens
- A3-size whiteboard and pens
- Post-it notes
- fidgeting material – Blu Tack, artist's rubber, origami paper
- audio technology options

### Takeaways from Chapter 8

- be aware of the poor working memory, make allowances
- embrace lots of fun, multi-sensory strategies
- encourage creativity
- focus on organization for homework and study

## CHAPTER NINE

# Helping with Homework

'How do they get time? How do they get their homework done so quickly? I'm still stuck inside. I wouldn't get time to myself. All my friends would be out playing and I'd still be inside.'

Abbie

## Dealing with Homework from the Early to Teenage Years

This chapter will provide various strategies and support options to help your child with homework from the primary years to secondary school. It looks at the specific challenges for the dyslexic child, and how you can help by:

- being understanding of the challenges
- creating the right stress-free environment
- not being a teacher at home
- communicating with school

If there is any particular chapter a dyslexic child will want a parent to look at, it's this one. The most significant issue for the parent and dyslexic child is confronting the schoolwork to complete at home. You are probably well aware why your dyslexic child is urging you to get to this chapter and heed any advice!

Homework is the biggest challenge for you and your dyslexic child, in terms of your relationship and whether your child experiences feelings of success or failure. There is such a fine line, a fine balance, between your child needing your help but then not wanting your help. You want to be able to create a calm, supportive environment for homework and study, and yet invariably you are reduced to nagging, shouting and constant clashes.

You really want to help and not cause more stress than is already there for your dyslexic child but, with the best intentions, it doesn't always work out as you'd hope. Both parties become frustrated, irritated and tired.

Let's look at the early years when young children are introduced to the notion of homework. You are so keen to be supportive for your young child, to the point where you are doing the homework for her.

## The challenges in the Early Years

'Very stressful, very difficult, the most stressful time doing homework because they were so tired and there was so much of it and everything took so long.'

Yvonne, parent, remembering homework in the primary years with three dyslexic sons

There is a lot to contend with, so we shall focus on key areas of difficulty and where you can help your child.

## Why is homework taking so long?
As already explored in earlier chapters, the mechanics of reading, writing and spelling and trying to process the information will affect the

time taken to complete homework. It all takes time. Distractions and avoidance tactics could also add to the hours it takes to do homework. How demoralizing for the child who is already exhausted after a challenging day in school, then to be confronted with more of the same at home.

> 'I have a lot, sometimes two hours . . . I feel tired. When my sister finishes before me, I feel cross, she gets to go and play.'
>
> Anna, 9

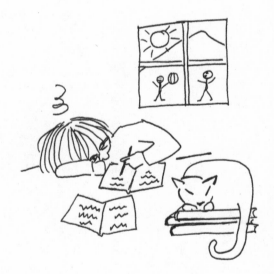

## How you can help

Liaise with the class teacher – make sure the school is aware how long your child is taking to complete homework compared to other pupils. And negotiate for your child to do less, but without 'dumbing down' content.

> 'I only have to do half of it.'
>
> Luca, 10

'They'd say do half an hour on English and Maths and I'd take two and a half hours. The teacher didn't believe I did a half-hour so my mum wrote a note to confirm I did the half-hour and she timed me.'

Caoimhe, remembering homework at primary school

<u>Make sure you have a stopping point, allowing time to play</u> – It is demoralizing for the dyslexic child to have to forfeit playing with friends because she needs more time to complete the homework she's been given. There needs to be encouragement, motivation and rewards for small successes.

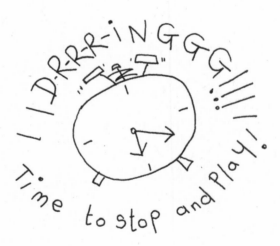

<u>Just stop!</u> – if the homework is taking a lot longer than anticipated by the teacher, and is resulting in exhaustion for the child and frustration for the parent, then it's time to stop. Put a note in the homework journal for the teacher to be aware of your child's struggle to complete her homework in the recommended time.

'If it takes more than one and a half hours, then stop. Homework was the worst time of the day and I'd have no time to play. It took three hours and a lot of tantrums all the way through.'

Roan, 11

You may also be dealing with a perfectionist who insists on completing all pieces just like everyone else. And who can blame your very determined dyslexic? Just be prepared for a lot of fractious moments and tiredness.

### Offer to read parts of the homework to save some time

'What helped a lot was Mum would read out the text and the questions and I would then grasp it easier. Mum acted as a reader.'

Jennifer

You can take some pressure off your already very tired child by offering to do the general tasks such as reading the questions or copying out the sums. It will save some time and energy and can be a relief for the child who struggles to read and copy down work.

## Does homework need to be so stressful?

You need to be aware how difficult homework can be for a dyslexic child – the simple tasks of copying, reading and spelling, which other children may take for granted, are all part of the challenges your child has to face. And remember, there will be good days and bad days – one day the homework will flow, while another day it will drag and everything learnt previously will be forgotten.

'Parents need to understand – they literally can't do it! Look at the page and imagine not being able to read it and how frustrating that is, and see from their perspective. The main thing is to be open about it and understanding.'

Molly's advice

**151**

<u>Be aware, be understanding</u> – remember, your child is tired after a day in school; all that concentrating, reading, writing, spelling, and quite probably several negative experiences. The thought of having to face more of the same at home will understandably bring avoidance tactics, refusal, tears and frustration. It is a very stressful time for both of you.

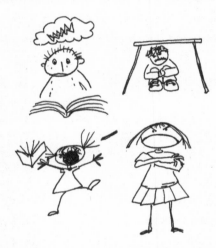

If you are also dyslexic then you will probably recognize these stresses from your own experiences, but that does not always mean you will have more patience! You will just get stressed over the dreaded homework together.

Do try to make allowances for a reluctance to do homework and the exhaustion that comes with it.

Dyslexics have to work on average four times harder than others to achieve.

'He'd come home absolutely exhausted from school, so I'd let him play and loosen up and relax before homework.'

Kate, parent

'The main challenges are that it will take a dyslexic twice as long to do homework compared to a child without dyslexia, and they might lose patience and concentration more often than not. Parents may feel frustrated with their child sometimes because it might take them longer, but it is important for parents to remember that if they are feeling a certain way, imagine what their child feels like! The main advice would be to support them with their homework and help them to figure out an answer.'

Nicola's advice

## Help . . . but don't help

This can be the most stressful part of doing homework as a dyslexic child – when is your help useful and appreciated, and when is your help interfering and time-wasting?

'They'd sit beside me and do my work with me, but then that would get infuriating. I'd want help but then I'd refuse help!'

Roan, 11

Initially, you have to help your young child with the concept of homework, but the aim right from the beginning is to increase independence. The best intentions can create tension at home, but there are small ways you can help your child without being seen to be overly involved.

Ideally, be available if required, but don't assume responsibility for the completion of homework. Help by not helping – if she is avoiding completing homework, then you must let her experience the consequences from school. And if she is struggling with a particular part of the homework, <u>don't do it for her</u>. The teacher needs to know those struggles are there.

'I used to get bad with homework – refused to do it.'

Luca, 10

**153**

'You've got to communicate with school. It's just not an option – all the tears and shouting at home. Two hours of homework and the parents are doing the homework! Don't do homework for them. The teacher is marking the parent instead of the child. Be around but don't do it for them.'

Danielle's advice as a parent

## Don't be a teacher at home.

Don't launch into a spelling or reading lesson with your child when all he is asking is how to spell or read a word. Do what is asked and no more. If you keep going into teacher mode he will stop asking!

'Follow what the child says when it comes to help – the child will know. Don't be constantly coming back and saying, "Oh, I can read this for you now!" You've done your bit, you can go now!'

Abbie's advice

'Prepare to be asked to spell words a lot! Don't look over their shoulder the whole time, but stay around and just prod them along if they're losing focus.'

Ben's advice

'It constantly bugs me my mum thinks I haven't read all the pieces in a Maths or English question. She reads over it and moves me out of the way of what I'm working on, and I'm fine. I could have been halfway through it by now. And she says, "Are you sure this one is right and are these spellings correct?" That's the teacher's job!'

Helena

If a piece of homework is causing particular trouble for your child then it is a good idea to put a note in his homework journal for the teacher to see he hasn't quite grasped this concept yet, and hopefully the teacher will plan a review lesson.

**154**

........................................

Remember, homework is always your child's responsibility, not yours.

........................................

And <u>never</u> take it upon yourself to give extra work over the holidays or weekends in the hope or belief that extra English instruction will make it all better. Your child is actually then being punished for something she cannot help. A long week in school and two hours of homework a day is hard enough, without parents adding to it all. Everyone deserves a break, and the holidays are a time when your dyslexic child can explore and enjoy her interests and strengths and not be reminded of her failings.

'My parents used to make me do English word books, extra work in the holidays, and I was crying. I just couldn't do it.'

Molly

'They help me, but sometimes they don't, they annoy me.'

Anna, 9, sums up parents helping at home very succinctly

## Make sure there are frequent, short breaks

All the reading and writing is hard work, so short breaks will give your child a boost and hopefully help motivation.

'I would advise parents to really understand how their child learns best and try to tweak the homework time to suit this. Short sessions per topic would be ideal. That being said, there will be times where there are very long homework sessions and heartache for all involved. Be calm, don't get frustrated. Be encouraging, not critical. Set targets and rewards, like a ten-minute break.'

Luke's advice

Some possible options for a short break:

- going for a walk
- having a kick around with a ball
- playing with the pet dog, cat or other pets
- getting a drink or a snack

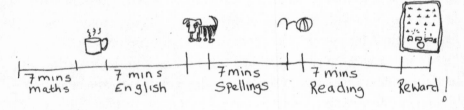

| 7 mins maths | 7 mins English | 7 mins Spellings | 7 mins Reading | Reward! |

## Create the right environment

'The key is: don't panic! And do not get frustrated with your child. Be patient. Homework time, especially primary, can be stressful. Make it a calm environment. Take one subject at a time. Praise your child when they do well.'

Emma's advice

'I like somewhere quiet. My mum helps with the first sum and checks I know what to do.'

Helena

Are you one of many parents who have their children doing homework in the kitchen, because it is easier for you to help at any moment and keep an eye on what they are doing? Be careful!

Apart from the fact you may be getting too involved and not encouraging self-reliance, the kitchen is not usually a quiet, calm space free from distractions.

Get out of the kitchen as soon as possible, certainly by the time your child is ten years old. Try to create a calm, quiet space for him, away from the communal area, so as to be an independent learner. Try to create gentle lighting that is not too bright, give shelving for books, and a desk or table where all equipment needed is easily accessible. This seems easy in theory but, in practice, you know there will still be frustrations and stresses at times. At least offering a calm space will go towards making homework a little less stressful for you and your child.

Here is some advice from parents who have been through the challenges of homework with their dyslexic children:

> 'Remove distractions for the child, but also remove yourself, so the session is as calm as possible. You need to be alert to pick up any difficulties as some things need to be explained in multiple ways before they can fully get the facts.'
>
> Liz

> 'I would read some of the pages with him to help him and take the pressure off him.'
>
> Mary

> 'Take time, be patient, be positive.'
>
> Lisa

> 'Routine is very important. Parents should stay calm and be patient and encourage all the time. I have an understanding with the school that if the workload is too much I can sign off on something.'
>
> Therese

## Why Is Being Organized Such an Effort?

If you have already looked at Chapter 8, you will know how a poor short-term memory affects a dyslexic child. Becoming a good organizer will be a huge help for this forgetful student.

In the primary school years, your child may forget to write down the homework, forget books, forget how to do the work, and just generally forget everything on top of the information overload from the school day. You need to instil good organization skills into your child as early as possible, as well as being supportive and offering a helping hand where necessary. This is not easy if you are also dyslexic and your own forgetfulness causes difficulties with organization.

### Help with preparations at the start of the homework session

A good idea is to make sure your child is set up to start the homework. Check she has all the homework written down correctly. Sometimes, a dyslexic child won't get the homework copied down fully from the board, so a good idea is to ask the class teacher to check that your child has all the correct details written down. Having a friend who can be relied upon to pass on any of the missed information is also very handy.

In the earlier years, your child may need you just to go through some of the instructions with her and to check she has all the material she needs. Then leave her to it as much as possible, being aware of time and suggesting breaks. Your child may not be aware of how much time the homework is taking.

You could give some useful materials to your child, including eraser pens, coloured paper and a whiteboard. A noticeboard on the wall can help focus and remind the dyslexic child of what there is to be done. Dyslexics need an overview and a plan, otherwise they can get quite overwhelmed and stressed. (See more on this in Chapter 10 and studying for exams.)

'My mum used to sit down with me and go through what I needed to do.'

Aoife, 13, remembering her early homework years

Emphasize the benefit of learning organization skills as early as possible in your child's school career. If your child relies too much on your constant reminders he isn't going to find ways to remind himself. Of course, if you are also dyslexic then you could be equally forgetful and disorganized. In that case, you probably have ways of your own to remember day-to-day things. Pass these on to your dyslexic child. And if you are not dyslexic you need to have the understanding that your dyslexic child has a poor working memory, which affects his organization and learning processes. He can't help it – so be patient.

'It may help for parents to set up a routine when their child comes home to do homework. It may help to do the following:

(i) set up a specific area for homework to be done;
(ii) dedicate the same time every day to do homework;
(iii) and make sure that the environment is quiet.

It is important for parents not to do the homework for their child. They need to be encouraging and to remind their child that they are doing great!'

Nicola's advice

## How Can Homework Be a Positive Experience?

Home learning is important but you have to question its value when it can create such unnecessary stresses for the dyslexic child, and fuels the feeling of incompetence for an already fragile self-esteem.

'It would take me hours . . . I'd come home crying about my work. Teachers would make the work slightly easier for me so then I'd just feel stupid.'

Roan

It can be an incredibly demoralizing time for young dyslexics, struggling in school and then struggling with homework, too, not receiving positive feedback for all their hard work.

'I could do it myself, but then I couldn't do it myself, and that really bugged me. I needed my mum to read it for me otherwise I wouldn't understand it. Loads of people were doing their homework themselves. I was struggling and it was really hard.'

Aoife

Apart from all the homework, students need to review work they have been learning in school, and that is even more important for the dyslexic with a poor working memory. But the rest of it – is it that valuable, we must ask ourselves?

'Homework is an overload for my daughter. She would be better off with less homework, as she does not learn from it, and more time to study through charts, stories, etc.'

Margaret, parent

If we consider some countries with very little homework, such as Finland, that are ranking high in most educational league tables, we have to question the value of some homework assignments – the stress, the grief they cause for the whole family. What is being achieved here when children feel under pressure to complete work to the best of their ability, only to be given mediocre marks for all their effort?

So don't forget to point out their unique talents and abilities, their ways of looking at the world and their strengths, despite and because of their dyslexia. That is a far more important role for you than being a teacher at home.

## The Challenges in the Secondary School Years

The fine balance between being supportive and being too involved with homework really reaches its crescendo in the teenage years. You can see that your dyslexic older child is struggling but you are in a frustrating position where he doesn't want your help and yet is in desperate need of help.

The greatest help from you would be to focus on one or two areas where you can make a difference, but otherwise you need to step back – stay away!

These are the areas where you can make a difference in the secondary school years:

- organization
- supplying useful material
- communicating with the school

## Transition from Primary to Secondary School Homework

Moving from primary to secondary school is a huge transition for any child but can be a particularly overwhelming experience for a dyslexic child. Suddenly the child is confronted by:

- a huge variety of different subjects
- having to move to different classrooms for each subject
- having to remember all the textbooks and exercise books for each subject
- lots of listening and note-taking of new subjects and new vocabulary
- having to make sure the homework is written down correctly before it's removed from the board
- a heavier homework load, where the content is unfamiliar territory

'What do they expect of me? You're faced with a lot of work pretty soon on, there's a lot of being overwhelmed. How am I supposed to do all this homework? When before I was doing just half an hour every evening, and now I'm stuck doing two hours, between six and seven subjects and I don't really know what I am doing!'

Mike, remembering going into
secondary school

'I'm always catching up. It just piles up.'

Roan

No wonder the dyslexic child is absolutely exhausted by it all and completely demoralized.

## How you can help

### Help your dyslexic get organized – in their own study space
If they haven't already moved from the kitchen to a study space to do their homework, then transition to secondary school is the time. You have to let go, however hard that may be. You won't be doing your older child any favours by allowing a reliance on you at this stage.

'After primary school they don't want you standing over them.'

Yvonne, parent

### Help with your child's homework environment
(See also Chapter 8 – getting organized with a poor working memory.)

Here are some ideas on how you can help create the right environment:

- aim for a personal study space free from distractions
- a desk or a table which can be left with book piles, Post-it note

reminders, and all equipment easily accessible, such as pens, highlighters, flashcards, a dictionary and thesaurus

- if possible, shelving space available for textbooks and subject folders
- the walls are free for Post-it reminders, the timetable, etc.
- a whiteboard or cork board for reminders and as a way to communicate something you want your teenager to remember
- offer equipment that will encourage organization of loose bits of paper and subject notes – box files, folders, file dividers, sticky labels
- if forgetting books at school or at home is a constant issue, colour code textbooks and exercise books in each subject, and have two sets of textbooks – one set for home and the other set for school
- help your older child to become more aware of the time it is taking to complete homework

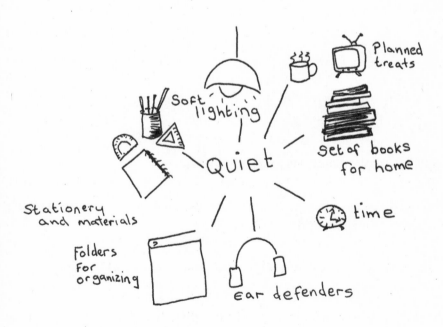

**CASE STUDY**

**JULIETTE, ON TACTICS SHE HAS USED FOR SECONDARY SCHOOL**

'I got a desk in my room. That was exciting, so much better. I could feel more responsible for my stuff. I had a section for my books and spare copies. The biggest issue for ages was all the different teachers and rooms and homework. Organization is a big issue – your bag has to be prepared. I got by with circular stickers for the corner of my books. All my Geography stuff would be red, History was green. I still know them off by heart. If I ran out of colours, then I would have a different pattern. I still use this system, Maths is blue, and my timetable is corresponding blocks of colour.'

'Have a whiteboard – I'd write down what I had to do – so Mum could see when a test is coming up and homework to do. Have sticky notes everywhere and a pin-board. Even with homework down in your homework journal, you forget.'

Alannah's advice

<u>Help your dyslexic maintain a daily routine</u>

You want your older child to be able to deal with all that secondary school throws at them, so encourage a daily routine and a sense of feeling in control for your child.

Feeling in control will help with the stresses and ups and downs of school.

- Encourage a routine for clearing out the school bag daily and packing it at night for the following day.
- Make sure the homework journal is being used at all times – it is

crucial with a poor short-term memory that everything is noted in the homework journal.

- If forgetting sports gear, instruments and so on occurs frequently, then have another copy of the school timetable in a prominent position, such as in the kitchen where you can spot what's coming up and give a reminder.

'I have photocopied timetables to ensure they are specific to my daughter, and labelled books with a specific colour per subject and set routines to help her cope with the more complicated aspects of time management in secondary school. This seems to have helped a lot but, as with anything one does, it is only obvious what is not working through failure. So as she isn't failing now, I choose to believe that the things we have done are working.'

Cathal, parent

Encourage self-reliance from the start, and just be supportive when it comes to organization. Practical advice and help will go a long way. Give guidance in setting up a routine, and encourage an increased confidence in their own ways of learning. The first term can be particularly challenging but they soon settle into their new environment and routines.

And remember, it is not laziness or carelessness on their part but a genuine struggle with organizational skills (and it's worth reminding the teachers of that!). So give understanding and positive support where you can, rather than nagging and criticism.

No teaching at home, stay away – consider an outside influence.

'I don't think the parent should be involved in homework at all.'

Danielle, parent

## Consider a specialist tutor

If possible, involve outside assistance, a specialist tutor who can be the one nagging your teenager and getting away with it. Your local Dyslexia Association should have a list of trained tutors for your area, or there may be college graduates, retired teachers and so on who can come to your home to help organize homework and study.

'Having a tutor, outside help – it was such a relief. You need somebody skilled. They're getting the skills how to do homework and study in school and outside. Parents aren't able to do that, you completely clash. That's the first step – learning the skills. If they go to a professional to learn the skills, that's a great help. You can't do that for them, they don't want you there.'

Yvonne, parent

## The option of a homework club

'Homework clubs are brilliant . . . saves the clash at home.'

Danielle, parent

There are certainly positives to homework clubs after school for students who are easily distracted. But as we know from earlier chapters, a dyslexic learner achieves more through multi-sensory learning, and therefore may need to move around, listen to music, talk through the work or fidget. And the quiet, regulated group environment does not encourage these more creative ways of learning.

'I like to listen to music to calm me. I can go to my own world where no one can interrupt.'

Sean, 13

## Supporting a Teenager through Secondary School

As time goes on and the work becomes more challenging, your dyslexic teenager may appreciate some help. The exhaustion and time spent doing homework can be eased if you give the help that is being requested – nothing more. But it is a fine balance!

'Mum always asks if I need help. She asks me questions on what I'm learning. Testing me helps. I like reading it out to my mum and she says it's good and is very impressed. But when I need to be left alone, leave me alone, don't be at me!'

Aoibhinn, 14

'Sit down with me for an hour if I need it. You need someone to guide you at times on your path, but you still need to make mistakes. Parents should be a back-up, a resource of knowledge and experience to help the student but not a force to pound in more school work . . . "You need to learn that, get this done . . ." etc.'

Mike's advice

'It's annoying – my parents would try to check my homework. They need to trust you and leave you to it. Don't come and check the homework every night. The teacher will check anyway. I like school to be my own thing, that I organize myself. A good idea is to remind the dyslexic what they need. The teacher would assume I didn't do it and give me a bad note, it would drive me insane. So tick off what I did in my journal. It's hard to be organized but it really helps. It is frustrating when you spend so long getting organized and then forget something.'

Juliette

'I try to continue an interest in all the subject areas my daughter is doing but increasingly get pushed off. This is a problem common to all parents, especially when kids turn to teens, but it is important somehow to engage to ensure that all is well in each subject.'

Cathal, parent (although his daughter may have a different way of looking at it!)

You just want to make life easier for your child who is spending too many hours trying to complete homework. Observe what works for them and go with it. Give them any materials they feel they need and, if you can find alternative ways for them to access information and present their work, then great.

As explored in other chapters, assistive technology can preserve energy levels that are usually used up in the mechanics of reading, writing and spelling.

## Communicate with school

Embrace one of your most useful roles – being an advocate for your child. Communicate with school if homework is taking too long, causing anxiety and unnecessary stress for your teenager. Negotiate with the school and subject teachers if possible.

Find alternative ways for your older child to produce homework such as an audio recording or typed essays. And remind teachers how dyslexia actually manifests for your dyslexic teenager; it's not just a spelling difficulty at this stage, far from it.

## Encourage self-belief

And what about all those red pen marks and poor results after the effort your teenager has taken over her homework? Self-esteem rapidly diminishes if homework is given negative feedback, despite the time and effort the dyslexic student has put into it. We all need to be reminded at times how much more effort the dyslexic student has to make to achieve the same as her peers.

This is where your other vital role comes in – encouraging self-belief and a strong self-esteem for your beleaguered dyslexic child. Support and encourage. Don't focus on the negatives or the poor subjects, but encourage the strengths, the stronger subjects, the unique abilities of the dyslexic mind. (See Chapter 12 for more on how you can foster self-belief.)

## Home Tools to Support Homework

### Equipment for the homework space
- eraser pens, highlighters
- whiteboard, cork board
- files, folders, file dividers
- coloured stickers, Post-its
- desk or a table, free from distractions
- gentle lighting, a side lamp
- shelving for books and folders
- copy of school timetable in the kitchen
- second set of textbooks
- communication via the homework journal

### Takeaways from Chapter 9

- be understanding of the challenges for your dyslexic child
- liaise with school to accommodate any difficulties
- help create the right environment
- know when to step back

## CHAPTER TEN

# Studying for Exams

'Understand what we're going through. It isn't a terrible thing, but it's not the best either! Oh, the joys of it all! So understand that it does take us longer to learn, and don't be pressuring us because that doesn't help at all!'

Abbie

## Supporting a Dyslexic Teenager

This chapter will offer advice on how you can best support your dyslexic teenager when it comes to studying and exams. It looks at the stresses of studying, and how you can help by:

- being understanding about the difficulties
- encouraging different study strategies
- stepping back

This is the chapter that may well elicit a very different response from the dyslexic teen compared to the parent who is keen to help. You may feel this is one of the most important chapters for you to take in, as you are eager to support your teenage dyslexic, and concerned that study time and study techniques are not going well. There is an added urgency if your dyslexic teenager is complaining of not being able to take in information or retain anything from her studies.

Your dyslexic teenager, on the other hand, would rather you skipped this chapter and left her to it! And if there are two points she wants you take from this chapter, they are: (i) <u>listen to what I need</u>; and then (ii) <u>step back</u>!

You may dismiss such advice, but do consider the contributions in this chapter from teenage dyslexics who feel that well-meaning but irritating parents add to their stresses!

---

**CASE STUDY**

**ABBIE WANTS TO BE SELF-RELIANT**

'I know my mum always wants to help – it's part of her nature to help me and tries her best to help me, but sometimes she needs to leave me to do it because sometimes that's the best for the situation, to do it myself.

'Trust your child a bit more that they know what they're doing. If they need the help, then fine, but don't be on top of them all the time . . . "Oh, I can read this for you . . !"'

---

## The Challenges of Studying

Studying can be a challenge for any student but, with the added frustration of a poor working memory and slower processing speed, it can become insurmountable for the dyslexic.

As explored in earlier chapters, difficulties with taking in written information, the ability to take productive notes, and then to memorize and retain these facts for an exam are huge challenges for a dyslexic student. They are sensitive to information overload because of their weak working memory, and could be so disheartened that they just give up.

### The main challenges for the dyslexic student

- the effort that goes into reading interferes with comprehension and memorizing
- processing information needs time
- inadequate notes are hard to follow
- poor organization and concept of time
- learning information by heart is very difficult due to poor working memory
- dyslexic difficulties increase with stress and tiredness
- feelings of frustration and failure
- complete exhaustion

> 'You're in school for such a long time, and then come home and do all your homework and study . . . where is there time to sleep?!'
>
> Caoimhe

Young people with dyslexia want parents to be aware of the particular issues they have to cope with when trying to study. They really don't need you to add to their stresses – they have enough with the frustrations of a poor short-term memory and the impossible task of rote learning.

**CASE STUDY**

**ADVICE FROM ABBIE**

'My mum goes through phases – "Oh yes, whatever you need to do . . ." – and then other times – "Will you just get on with it! Just get it done! You've been on this for an hour!"

'Don't be constantly nagging! Try to accept what we do to help ourselves and not nagging us and herding us on. There's no need for two of us to get stressed! Try to keep calm. My mum is stressed for the both of us!

> 'No matter what, my mum would always lose her cool at some stage. I know she reads all the books but she never really fully understands what it's like to be dyslexic. If you're not dyslexic, you won't actually understand fully what we go through or how hard it can be sometimes.'

Parents can exacerbate the situation if they lack an understanding of how a dyslexic prefers to learn or an awareness of the added challenges for their dyslexic child that other non-dyslexic children may not experience. Be aware and make allowances.

## How you can help your dyslexic teen with these challenges

Don't nag! If you tell a teenager to study, invariably that is the last thing that will happen!

> 'Just because you told me to study, I'm not going to do it. It is annoying. Because you said it, I'm not going to do it now.'
>
> Áine

Naturally, it can be difficult to stop yourself from telling a reluctant teenager to study, but you need to make allowances for extreme tiredness after a day in school, as well as the frustration of knowing that hours of study won't get the results they want and deserve.

Back off! This can be hard to accept if you are quite hands-on and involved with your child's education attainments. But if you want to avoid clashes and truly support your dyslexic teen with her studies, then respect her space, back off and just be there if needed. Try to be calm and give space, while letting your teenage dyslexic know that you are there if needed – a difficult balance.

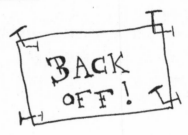

'If somebody was always at me I'd be flustered and all over the place and I'd feel all up in a heap, and then I wouldn't be able to get stuff done because I'd be angry and all over the place. As long as my mum knows I'm working away, and knows I'm doing the best I can.'

Róisín

There are more productive, practical ways you can support your dyslexic teenager who needs to study.

## Four Main Strategies for Improved Studying

1. help to create a study environment
2. support a variety of study techniques
3. help with the concept of time
4. be supportive around exam time

### Create the right study space

'You want to make it comfortable for them – as long as it's their choice how they study. No distractions – a designated area for study, away from games.'

Sean

The issue with a study space will depend on what individual students prefer as a study environment, whether complete quiet or perhaps music and background noise to aid concentration. Either way, try to give them whatever they find conducive for their study space.

> 'I like spinning round in my chair and I listen to music – I don't like being in a quiet room. They don't really work for me.'
>
> David

The main thing is that there is the offer of a calm space that can be called their own, where they can access their textbooks, notes and Post-it reminders without disruption.

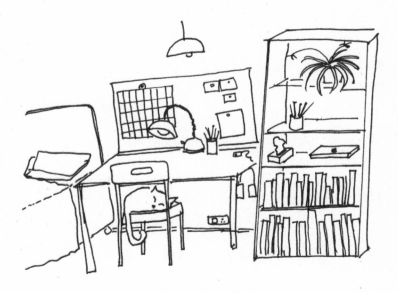

> 'Leave my study space to me, I know where things are. My dad used to come in and clear it and then I couldn't focus, I didn't know what to do.'
>
> Tadhg

Provide the stress-free space and leave them to it!

> 'What I love about having a desk and my own room is I can keep it my own way and have things organized the way I need. I find it faster if I can just sit down and do it on my own.'
>
> Helena

And if you would like to help in any way with their study space, then offer to provide some useful stationery and equipment to encourage organization of subjects and study notes. They may also appreciate initial help with sorting papers into subject folders. In their own words, dyslexic students can tell you what equipment really helps them:

> 'A calendar on the wall helps me be organized.'
>
> Leah

> 'Flashcards, coloured pens and paper and folders, so I can organize myself.'
>
> Claire

> 'I like white flashcards and different-coloured pens.'
>
> Áine

> 'Pads, pull-out pages, and small pads to write things down.'
>
> Ewan

> 'Coloured paper is always handy and loads of different highlighters.'
>
> Emma

> 'I love having the whiteboard and all my folders. I have a folder for each subject. I use a small chalk board for taking down mind-maps and for doing Maths.'
>
> David

Chapter 8 and Chapter 9 give you further ideas on how you can help create a study environment for your dyslexic child.

## Be open to a variety of study ideas

'I'm good at mind-maps. I didn't know that before. I can visually see, and I know I have to hear myself say it or write it. I know I can't just read it. It really helps – knowing how I learn.'

Alex

All children learn differently, and you now know that finding his own individual learning style is invaluable for a dyslexic child. Your studying teenager can emphasize his stronger learning channel and also be multi-sensory to help process and memorize information.

'I would advise parents to really understand how their child learns best.'

Luke

It is really important that when it comes to study you are aware of the short-term memory issue, and that more unconventional ways of studying could be beneficial for your dyslexic teen. Do some research on multi-sensory learning, encourage the dyslexics in your family to do questionnaires online to find out what kind of learner they are, such as www.vark-learn.com.

Go to study skills seminars and talks with your dyslexic teenager. Be aware of the variety of ways to learn and retain information out there. Anything that will offer strategies that could suit your teen's learning preferences, whether visual, auditory or kinaesthetic / tactile, will be worth exploring.

'Look out for courses, events and seminars to find out new ways to learn and meet other parents with dyslexic teenagers. Help by getting websites for various organizations and any multi-sensory techniques.'

Claire

All students benefit from study skills and knowing how to be an effective learner, and dyslexic students need more guidance than others to develop these skills. Training in study skills is a good idea, and these techniques can be introduced and taken on and adapted or not – allow flexibility. If possible, get one-to-one help for your dyslexic child with a specialist in dyslexia and multi-sensory learning. This tutor will be able to help your child find his learning strengths and offer a variety of strategies to approach his studies.

The main thing is to be open to unexpected ways of learning. Don't assume that reading or writing something over and over again will make it stick, and let your struggling teenager know that, too.

'They need to remember this is our way of learning and, in the long run, it will be faster learning this way rather than doing it their way – like reading it over and over is just ridiculous!'

Abbie

It is OK to do things differently, let them explore ways of working that will use their dyslexia constructively. Encourage finding their own personal learning style, what works best for them. They don't have to do things the way everyone else does, which also means do not compare how they study with non-dyslexic siblings.

'My mum would say, "Why can't you study like that?" But I can't. Don't compare your children. My sister gave me her old notes but we learn in completely different ways, so I didn't use her things. She used mind-maps in Science . . . I said, "Get away from me!"'

Caoimhe

## Help with multi-sensory study strategies

(More on multi-sensory learning can be found in Chapters 6, 8 and 9.)

### Visual

- get good film versions of studied texts for English studies
- provide a whiteboard, flashcards, coloured paper and pens
- provide lots of coloured paper and coloured A4 pads
- allow Post-its of quotes and definitions around the home

'Allow your child to put notes on the cupboards or wherever – important and short pieces of information on a cupboard door. I'd open a cupboard in the kitchen and see "enzymes".'

Niamh

### Auditory

- find out about assistive technology for audio versions of textbooks and notes
- get audio versions of studied texts in English and other subjects
- encourage them to give a mini lecture or talk about a topic to you
- allow them to work with music in the background if it helps concentration

'Listening to the plays I was studying proved extremely beneficial for my play Macbeth. This aural learning gave me an extra dimension as I learn very well that way and could recall multiple quotes from the play to this day.'

Luke

### Kinaesthetic / tactile

- be aware that this is usually the strongest learning channel for a dyslexic and invariably underused
- let them walk around and move about while learning if they prefer

- if they need to fidget to aid concentration, then so be it!
- provide Blu Tack, elastic bands, an artist's rubber, origami paper, or whatever is needed in order for the 'fidgeter' to concentrate

'My mum used to give out to me because I'd run around the table, run and run to learn something off. I'd run around in circles and I felt I was getting it, then my mum would tell me to stop and listen to what she's saying.'

Juliette

'Allow your child to do the opposite of what you think is right! If they need a pen in their hand to flick, let them do it!'

Tadhg

Ultimately, they have to find their own way. A variety of multi-sensory techniques will be the most beneficial, and will make studying more enjoyable for the otherwise stressed dyslexic student.

'Sometimes you can make it fun – be creative rather than just stuck in the book. My mum says, "Will you just hurry up and learn it . . . never mind your colours and all!"'
'My mum just wants the job done.'

Abbie

'If they want to fidget, let them fidget. Give them breathing space. Occasionally, I want to get up and walk around and recite it – so give me space to do that.'

John

'The hardest part about secondary school is study – don't question them about their methods of study – if it works for them, then it works for them. Don't make them doubt their own strategies if it's actually working.'

Good advice from Ewan, 13

## Help with time management

Make sure there are plenty of breaks.

> 'I need a lot of breaks to concentrate in my sessions, otherwise I just don't take it in.'
>
> Claire

Most students can be distracted and lose concentration when studying, but this is a serious issue for individuals with dyslexia. Be aware of a lack of focus after a relatively short period of concentrated work, and make sure lots of short breaks are built into your dyslexic child's study routine. Working for lots of short periods of time is so much better than sitting down solidly for two hours but not actually studying productively.

> 'Don't make them sit down for three hours straight! Let them go out for twenty minutes and then study for forty minutes. Let them have breaks.'
>
> Alannah

Good productive studying can be undertaken for 20-40 minutes, and then a short 5-10-minute break (to have a drink or snack, play with the dog, have some fresh air) will give the dyslexic brain a rest before returning to concentrated study.

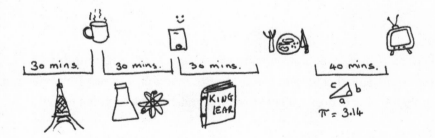

At the beginning, you could sit down with your dyslexic child and go through a realistic study timetable, with breaks and treats included if he needs that focus and motivation.

> 'The one sit-down chat – one big conversation about study rather than a lot of nagging. Sit down together and make the plan with plenty of breaks, and be understanding about little-and-often studying.'
>
> Aoibhinn

## Help organize time to review topics

Due to the poor working memory, the dyslexic student will need a lot of overlearning and frequent reviewing in some subjects. So encourage regular reviewing, little and often, of topics such as Science, History or Geography. Revision for exams becomes less daunting and easier to deal with when the dyslexic student is in the habit of regularly reviewing material. Consistent work through the term will be more beneficial than trying to cram everything at the last minute.

You could also help time efficiency by offering alternative notes, such as revision books with good summaries and bullet points, and alternative ways to produce revision notes, such as mind-mapping apps and audio technology. You could also offer to read texts for your dyslexic child, so she can focus on taking notes and learning.

> 'Dad would offer to read if I'm tired and it's getting late. He'd just offer in case.'
>
> Niamh

The main aim (in an ideal world) is to concentrate on learning and understanding throughout the year, with studying and regular reviewing, and not trying to attempt rote learning and cramming at the last minute.

> 'Be supportive – as much as the child may hate revising, they have to review, otherwise the words "I remember everything" will backfire!'
>
> Sean

## Help with exam preparation

### Focus on exam accommodations

Find out what special arrangements are available for your dyslexic teen in his state exams (if any). It will really help to reduce stress levels and give your teenager the chance to show his knowledge and abilities. Where are the application forms? What are the deadlines? Where do you need to sign? And make sure any reasonable accommodations are also being practised in all in-house exams. (See Chapter 11 on being an advocate at exam time.)

'It will help me show what I mean. If I was writing it, I'd be more conscious of time, but now I have a scribe it's her job to get it done. So I can concentrate on doing my best and not the spelling and grammar.'

Sarah, on being granted the opportunity to dictate her answers to a scribe

'I love it, having my own room and a reader. At first, I didn't like the idea of it but now I love it. It's such a big difference now . . . I don't see everyone turning pages and writing. I can be in my own zone and I can just focus on myself and my paper with no distractions.'

Jennifer, on being granted her own room and a reader for her state exams

### Encourage familiarity with exam papers

Planning the time allotted for each section of an exam paper can prove very difficult for a dyslexic student, so the opportunity to practise exam papers, either alone, with a parent or part of a group, would be very beneficial. Make sure to get past exam papers in a booklet or via the Internet for your dyslexic teenager to practise. It is a good way for them to familiarize themselves with the wording of questions and the timing. They will gain in confidence if they have plenty of practice with exam questions and checking sample answers.

### Don't add to their stress!

Your studying teen needs a complete break from study at some point in the week. Make sure your dyslexic child has one whole day off from studies, such as a Saturday, to be with friends and to relax. This is not avoiding study, this is allowing the brain to continue to process and integrate information already studied before taking on any new information.

> 'Do something completely different, do random stuff, change the subject completely, stop focusing on study. Go and do something like rollerblading!'
>
> Juliette

Allow them to go out to events at the weekend or to see friends, rather than virtually punishing them by insisting they do more studying because of their dyslexia. Yes, they need to get down to their studies, but they also need time to themselves, to rest their minds, and to have plans with friends that help reduce stress levels and boost motivation.

> 'Don't put on any pressure – give them time to go out and be with friends.'
>
> Katie

And encourage your stressed-out dyslexic to feel in control. Don't take over, however much you want to be involved. Encourage self-reliance and self-belief.

> 'I don't like to be asked questions on it. I don't like to talk about it too much, it stresses me more. Asking me how I'm doing is fine, but if my mum says, "You should do this . . . you should go over your science experiments," it just annoys me and I don't do it!'
>
> Maeve

'You can't do it for them, they don't want you there. Parents can't be a teacher, so they need to have the skills themselves.'

Yvonne, parent

## And finally – be supportive emotionally

One of your most important roles is, of course, to be there at times of disappointment when all your dyslexic child's hard work and effort are not reflected in her results.

Remember that 'success is in the effort', and don't over-focus on grades or comparisons with others. Sometimes, you just need to remind yourself how much more work your dyslexic teenager needs to put into exams to reach her potential and equal or exceed her peers.

'If they know you're behind them and supporting them, that makes a huge difference. Don't make a big deal about the dyslexia.'

Kate, parent

Often, they do not see themselves as successful students and can suffer from anxiety in the build-up to exams. Help to decrease stress levels, and recognize and praise hard work at a vulnerable time. Praise effort rather than results. Point out successes and encourage strengths.

'My mum reassures me and keeps me calm ... "Whatever you get you'll have tried your hardest."'

Emma

## Takeaways from Chapter 10

- be understanding of the challenges for a dyslexic student
- be open and encouraging of alternative ways to study
- don't add to the stresses
- be supportive emotionally

## CHAPTER ELEVEN

# Communicating with School and Being an Advocate

'I would say the parent has to be an advocate the minute they suspect something is up. Then when the whole process starts you have to keep being the voice asking everything and pushing, because who else is going to?'

Niamh, parent

## Critical Support throughout a Child's School Career

This chapter will look at how best to support your dyslexic child at crucial points in your child's school career. It looks at the parent's role as an advocate from the early years to the final exams, by:

- knowing your child's rights
- being prepared
- communicating and negotiating
- making informed decisions

Being an advocate for your child is a vital role in terms of generating the full array of support you want for your dyslexic child who is struggling in school. Your new-found knowledge of dyslexia will help you to be confident and determined in dealing with the education system. No one is going to care about your child quite as much as you do, so you will often find yourself liaising with school and making sure everything is in place to support your dyslexic child, and that these support structures remain in place.

## The Beginning of the Journey

Your role as an advocate for your child starts before the word 'dyslexia' is even mentioned, as explored in Chapter 3 (see advice on obtaining an educational psychologist's assessment for your child and pursuing any recommendations). As soon as you feel that your child is struggling with conventional teaching methods, you begin on a sometimes tortuous path, making sure your child receives fair and equal access to opportunities within the education system.

> 'What parents should expect: hard work and worry! The educational system is using just one way of learning and we have to help our children in any way to help them get the most out of the system, and if that means going head to head with the system, so be it. Demand the best and hopefully you'll get it.'
>
> Elmarie's advice as a parent of a dyslexic daughter

### Know your rights

....................................................

Children with dyslexia have the right to equal access to education, the chance to learn in a style that suits their way of processing information and opportunities to show their capabilities.

....................................................

Along with your growing knowledge about your child's specific learning difference, make sure to take note of the latest Education Act on specific needs. An inclusive statement made by the Department of Education, which determines that the educational needs of all children are identified and provided for, will remind you of your child's rights. The school's mission statement will also help you determine your child's rights and the support he deserves.

This sounds like fighting talk but, unfortunately, you may find yourself at various points in your child's school career fighting for your child's needs to be met.

### Be prepared to fight

You may have to fight for services, fight for people to understand how your child learns, fight for basic awareness of dyslexia and, finally, fight with your own inner worries that you have not done enough for your child.

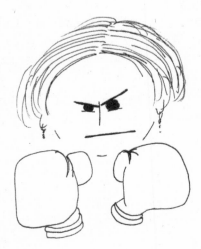

'My mother fought my cause on multiple occasions and I would not be in the same position today if it wasn't for her support. She got me tested and fought for support at my primary school. She sent me to extra classes, tutorials and dyslexia sessions. She fought for my spelling and grammar waiver for the state exams. She provided me with every opportunity she possibly could along the way.'

Luke, engineer

## Advocating during the Primary School Years

### Consider your expectations

Do not make assumptions that your child's school is equipped to accommodate the specific learning differences of a dyslexic child. Do not assume that all teachers and those working in learning support are fully up to date with the changing attitudes to dyslexia and how best to help a dyslexic child thrive in class.

If you have followed your gut feeling and pursued an assessment for your child through the school, you may well have experienced the frustrations of many parents of children with dyslexia. The specific difficulties of the dyslexic pupil are just not considered severe enough for an assessment or any offer of resource hours. School budgets are stretched; your child is doing 'all right' and therefore not considered a priority for any costly intervention. Combined with minimal awareness of dyslexia at a professional level, you feel exasperated by the lack of movement towards any appropriate support measures for your talented but struggling dyslexic child.

'It is very difficult for parents when schools do not have the know-how, the understanding or the budget to assist those with dyslexia. My experience in primary was that the teachers knew nothing about dyslexia, just always blamed my child. Dyslexia was never mentioned by the teachers as they knew they could not assist and did not have a budget to cover an assessment.'

Margaret, parent

Even after negotiating a professional assessment through the school, or paying for an educational psychologist working privately, you cannot be certain that your child will receive the level of support as recommended in the completed report.

'Communication is so important. Keep requesting resource time if you're not getting it. Expect nothing! Be willing to fight for your child if necessary!'

Brenda, parent

## Communicate regularly

Regular and positive communication with your child's school is central to your role as an advocate for your child, and will be a positive influence on her progress and the effectiveness of the school's actions on her behalf.

'Meet with the teachers at least once a term. They will know you are serious about your child. After problems start, get in there and make yourself known as soon as possible. They will realize that you are on board where your child's education is concerned and will gladly work with you.'

Elmarie's encouraging advice as a parent

Children with dyslexia learn differently and this needs to be understood and accommodated by your child's school. You can pass on to the school your own understanding of how your child prefers to learn, his abilities as well as his weaknesses. You cannot tell teachers how to do their job but there are areas where you can help to make a positive difference for your dyslexic child struggling at school.

Anything that causes unnecessary stress or feelings of low ability for the very aware dyslexic child should be open to negotiation with your child's teachers.

Possible areas for negotiation are:

- reading out loud in class
- writing out spellings on the board in front of the class
- number and difficulty of words in the weekly spelling tests
- amount of homework given per night
- alternative ways to produce creative writing, such as using assistive technology
- over-emphasis on rote learning, which requires a strong short-term memory

> 'Make teachers aware that being called up to the board is traumatizing when you're young and you can't spell the word, or when reading out loud. It's really important teachers are aware you won't be able to keep up with the spelling standards, but not that it affects your intelligence.'
>
> Katie's advice, from her own experiences in primary school

## Pursue appropriate resource hours or learning support

The emphasis is on <u>appropriate support</u> for your dyslexic child, who struggles with certain aspects of learning while having strong abilities in other areas (as shown in an educational psychologist's detailed report). You want the school to implement appropriate support as recommended in the report, while at the same time not wanting your child to feel excluded from class activities or stupid compared to his peers. It is a difficult balance and one you need to be aware of for the sake of your child's self-esteem.

> 'This is where the constant fight about balance starts. Yes, you want help for your child, but we don't want them to be separated or treated differently from their peers. There is a balance between special treatment and segregation. Kids aren't stupid and they know the difference. One-to-one sessions are welcomed by the child but integration remains important.'
>
> Cathal, parent

Communication and negotiation with your child's school are crucial when it comes to any individual education plan for your child. Keeping your relationship with school open and co-operative will help your cause. You can contribute to the development and implementation of your dyslexic child's learning support through regular discussion with the school via formal meetings and, possibly most productively, in informal chats.

> 'Resources are so limited in the education system that I believe that parents need to constantly be an advocate for their children. I spoke to my son's teacher at the beginning of the school year to understand what support classes he would receive, and to agree on areas that I would work on with my son as part of his homework on a daily basis.'
>
> Mary, parent

### Remind the school of your child's abilities

Make sure your child is not feeling inadequate compared to her peers because of a notion of low ability and work being 'dumbed down' for her to complete. She may actually enjoy reading out loud and opportunities to perform poetry or drama. She may enjoy writing stories and being asked challenging questions in class or difficult maths concepts. Her creative mind wants to be challenged.

> 'Trust your instincts. Don't let your child languish in a tiny resource class with no friends, being kept back doing simple work. Just be an advocate for your child and an advocate within school. You have to remind your child and the school on an ongoing basis that your child is not stupid. It's not something people learn once, you have to do it all the time.'
>
> Danielle, parent

## Don't be afraid to move schools if necessary

---

**CASE STUDY**

**CATHAL, PARENT, ADVISES THAT YOU SHOULD MAKE CHANGES IF NECESSARY**

'Listen. If your child is saying they are having difficulty with the way things are being taught, then it means that they want to learn but can't do it the way the teacher has defined. So find another way. Make changes if things aren't working. This is where it gets difficult. You must be aware and prepared to move your child if the school isn't doing what is necessary.

'In the first school, they thought they were helping but they didn't know what they were doing. My daughter was suffering. She is bright, witty and creative but they saw her as different, no good at English and hard to deal with academically. The second school saw her gifts and intelligence and found many ways to make her shine.'

---

If you sense that your child is feeling disheartened, upset and not enjoying school, then pay attention to what is going on in terms of how your child is being taught, what progress she is making and how support strategies are being incorporated into her learning programme.

Your child's self-esteem is your main concern. Finding a nourishing educational environment that suits your dyslexic child is your focus. Your best guide is your child, and seeing if she feels challenged in terms of her strengths and supported in the development of her weaker skills.

After the initial frustrations, you should be seeing your child progressing and growing in confidence. The primary school years can be very exposing for the dyslexic child. Consequently, you must be a sensitive and aware observer of your child's relationship with school, and be an advocate for your child when she is losing heart.

> 'Parents need to pinpoint what is going on and make sure to make life easier for you, for your sake.'
>
> Abbie's advice as a dyslexic pupil

## Choosing a Secondary School

Choosing the right school, where you feel your child will thrive, can be a stressful period of decision-making for a parent. Choices are often limited for parents when their dyslexic child is moving from primary to secondary school. Nevertheless, advice from parents who have already been through this process can be invaluable.

---

**CASE STUDY**

**KATE AND UWE ON CHOOSING A SECONDARY SCHOOL FOR THEIR DYSLEXIC SON**

Kate: 'We arranged meetings with schools and Mike was part of it himself. We researched and asked him what he would like. He'd be more motivated if he was included in the decision-making, if he felt he had more power over his life and he wasn't a victim of having dyslexia. Do the research with your child. Look at the availability of subjects and the support system in the school.'

Uwe: 'We actually went to a couple of schools with him, talked to teachers and the Principal and told them he was dyslexic. Here's the report. What is available at the school to support him?'

---

## Some guidance on choosing a school

- Gather information and get advice from other parents and your local branch of the Dyslexia Association. Their knowledge and experience will be invaluable.
- Arrange meetings with schools.
- Get a sense of each school's attitude to students with dyslexia – do they see them as having a learning difference or a learning disability?
- What subjects are offered?
- How do they place students in classes – streaming or mixed ability?
- To what extent is assistive technology available for students?
- Make sure your dyslexic child is part of the decision-making.

## A note on subject choices

Some subjects will be a huge challenge for a dyslexic individual, while other subjects will make more sense and offer the opportunity for success. Areas of strength could include the more practical subjects such as Technology, Home Economics or Engineering. The more logical, numerical subjects, such as Mathematics, Accounting and Business could also suit the dyslexic mind.

The creative dyslexic will be looking for a good Art department, and Music and Drama opportunities. And sometimes a dyslexic will have a great interest in languages and would like options such as Italian and Japanese.

Each dyslexic student will have his own strengths and interests. We cannot assume that if you are dyslexic you must be good at practical subjects.

> 'All dyslexics are different. I wasn't good at Art. It doesn't mean you are good at practical subjects.'
>
> Tadhg, 15

When a school offers a variety of subjects which demand creativity and problem-solving skills, you can be confident that your dyslexic child will find an area where he can progress well. The most important thing is that they make their own decisions on what subjects they would like to try.

> 'Parents shouldn't put any pressure on doing certain subjects. They shouldn't reflect themselves in their child, and the subjects they want them to do well in are their own favourite subjects. Respect the decisions your child is making.'
>
> Niamh's advice

## Streaming or mixed ability?

If you find a school you are interested in uses the process of streaming to place students in classes, then think twice about sending your dyslexic child into that system. Streaming will place your dyslexic child in a class based on his performance in an assessment test. This is not good news for an otherwise quite capable individual, who struggles to complete conventional tests within a specific time limit. Invariably, the dyslexic student will find himself in the lower-ability stream because he wasn't able to produce the accuracy and fluency required in the test for the higher stream. The lower-ability classes will cultivate a poor self-image, while failing to challenge the dyslexic or stimulate any of his strengths.

Mixed ability is what you will be looking for in a school's approach to placing students, where each class comprises children of varying abilities. A dyslexic will be at an advantage in a class where there are opportunities for the creative mind to be challenged in a variety of activities, and to contribute to class discussions.

If a school allows a dyslexic to languish in a lower-ability class then what is that saying about that school's attitude to learning differences?

'Entrance exams were really scary. Make the school aware about putting a dyslexic in the lower classes.'

Katie's thoughts on streaming

There will be no perfect school that will meet all your criteria, so you must decide what are the most important factors for you and your child that will support your child's progress.

## Handy Hints for Preparing for Secondary School

'Go into secondary school prepared . . . don't assume they will do it for you. Have your own knowledge of what you want to be done – like resource or dropping a language. Be firm in your decisions, be assertive from the beginning.'

Molly's advice to parents

As explored in earlier chapters, transition to secondary school can be a huge challenge for a dyslexic child who will be under the added pressure of a poor working memory. They are trying desperately to remember everything they are being told about this new place and its many rules, new subjects and teachers. Added to all that is the pressure to produce more demanding pieces of work and more developed answers, compared to primary school.

Being an advocate for your dyslexic child will be critical in that first term when the Principal, year head, subject teachers and resource teachers need to be informed of your child's difficulties and responsive to his needs.

**Make sure the school is aware of your child's educational needs**
Contact the resource staff – making contact with the resource or

learning support department will be beneficial for a smooth transition to secondary school.

> 'It is very important to ensure that I am getting the best help and support for my son to give him every opportunity to succeed as he enters secondary school. My son starts secondary school this year and I have met the resource team in his school in advance and reviewed my son's requirements with them.'
>
> Mary, parent

<u>Prepare a summary of your child's report</u> – it is easy to overlook the needs of individual students in a busy and demanding setting. You cannot assume that all the information relating to your child will be passed on to each of his teachers. A good idea is to present a synopsis of your child's educational psychologist's report, outlining the results and recommendations (no more than a one-page summary). This can be given to your child's subject teachers, while making sure that the Principal and the resource teachers have copies of the complete report.

Be aware that there will be some teachers who do not have the understanding of dyslexia that you now have, so be prepared to give details on how dyslexia manifests for your child. You may have to explain why reading out loud in class is stressful or that a poor working memory makes organization of school books challenging.

See Chapters 8, 9 and 10 on how you can help your child deal with organization, homework and studying at secondary school.

## Maintaining Support for a Teenage Dyslexic

It is your job to deal with the school on behalf of your older child as he manoeuvres through the secondary school system. You want your teenage dyslexic to have fair and equal access to educational opportunities.

'In secondary, it is a different story, they have too many children competing for the same resources. Get outside help, make yourself known to the teachers and advocate for any equipment that can help.'

Elmarie, parent

In an ideal world, the school will:

- be aware of the recommendations as found in the educational psychologist's report
- allow the use of assistive technology, such as audio versions of textbooks
- arrange for alternative notes in subjects
- make allowances for a poor working memory and difficulties with organization skills
- offer learning support in a one-to-one or small-group setting and assist with the more challenging subjects
- understand dyslexics have good days and bad days and pressure can make symptoms worse

However, as your dyslexic child progresses through secondary school, she is more likely to be taking more command of her educational progress, communicating her needs to the school on her own terms. Be sensitive and work behind the scenes to fight for equal opportunity for your dyslexic teenager. Make sure to involve her in any meetings and all decision-making. It is <u>her</u> school experience, after all.

'The child says, "This is what I need you to do," rather than the other way round and the parent telling the child what to do.'

Mike's excellent advice to parents

'What parents have to do would be all behind the scenes. I'd never want my parents to go in front of a class to talk to a teacher. I'd rather go and talk to the teacher myself. I'd always want to be in the meeting. I hate when people talk about me when I'm not there to give my opinion. I could express my needs better than my mum . . . she could never grasp it fully because she has never experienced it, but she does try.'

Tadhg, 15

'The homework journal is a good way to communicate.'

Yvonne's advice as a parent

## Parent–teacher meetings – how they offer you an opportunity

Parent–teacher meetings are sometimes the only opportunity you will have to meet with your child's teachers and highlight his needs as well as his abilities. You cannot assume that each teacher is aware of your child's dyslexia, so this will be a chance to let them know or to remind those who need reminding.

'Definitely always mention dyslexia at every parent–teacher evening. You need to talk to each teacher and speak each time. Tell each teacher, new teachers and trainees. You need to tell teachers about organization and memory difficulties. The teacher apologized, she wasn't aware. I thought she knew but she didn't know, and was very apologetic.'

Yvonne's advice as a parent of three dyslexic sons

'Parent–teacher meetings may be the only opportunity for parents to discuss dyslexia. Try to explain to the teachers, keep mentioning their dyslexia: "Yes, but he's dyslexic."'

Tadhg, 15

Sometimes you will need to educate teachers on how dyslexia has its strengths and that it is not a barrier to success. There is every possibility that a student with dyslexia can perform at the highest level in subjects such as English and Maths.

'If a teacher says something you don't agree with then speak up! If you know your child has potential and the teacher won't understand or doesn't agree, just tell your child to prove them wrong, like I did to my English teacher.'

Sarah, 15

Sometimes you are just going to have to push for your child's educational rights in that parent–teacher meeting.

'Be forceful and request extra study classes to go over particular subjects, hand-outs of notes, a scribe, audio versions of notes and so on. What can each teacher do for your child to best maximize your child's progress through school?'

Mike's advice

## How to Be an Advocate During Exam Time

### Keep up to date

Keep up to date with the latest developments in the education system. Options and criteria for exam support could keep changing for students with specific difficulties. And don't rely completely on the school to be aware of the latest developments.

'It's very important to get all the facts and information when it comes to the state exams. But it is also important to find out as much as you can about school work and entitlements and allowances. It is important to find out as much as you can about every aspect – the school, the impact on the child, everything you can possibly find out. It is important the parent keeps on top of things and keeps in touch and keeps fighting for all that is necessary, the allowances, and the support from teachers.'

Niamh's advice as a parent

There is a great deal of information out there, including changing regulations and technological advances. The latest information on exemptions from languages, exam accommodations and assistive technology can be found via relevant websites and your local dyslexia association. Gather any information that you feel will help your dyslexic child cope with the demands of the state exams. You want to ensure your teenager has equal opportunity and a smooth progression through the education system. Never assume your dyslexic teenager will be granted a spelling and grammar waiver or extra time in an exam. Check and double check.

## Appeal if necessary

If you feel aggrieved that your child has been refused the exam accommodations that you believe are his right (check the latest Education Act and the school mission statement), then appeal, appeal, appeal. Follow the process as offered by the Department of Education. Alternatively, lodge a complaint with the ombudsman, who examines complaints from members of the public who feel they have been unfairly treated by certain public bodies.

> 'They don't leave it up to the school, they know what needs to be done.'
>
> Áine, on her parents' input

## Keep records

It is really important that you keep written records of all your meetings with the school and other professionals. Maintain a folder where you can keep copies of all correspondence, along with all the professional reports completed by educational psychologists, occupational therapists, and so on. The school will have a file on your child and so should you. You need to be armed if you are going into battle!

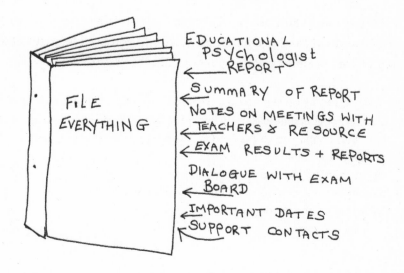

'Basically, that's the way things work – you really need to do it yourself. Keep files in a filing cabinet – any correspondence, reports, etc. Better to have a file so you have everything there then.'

Yvonne, parent

## Keep fighting

'Looking back, my parents had to fight my ground in my last few years of secondary school in regards to me getting extra support during my exams. My parents went and sought after an independent educational assessment. My school did offer assessments, but they were only offered to students with severe dyslexia. If it wasn't for my mum pushing for me to get one done, then I more likely than not wouldn't have received two out of the three waivers in my exams.'

Nicola

You want your teenager to have as much chance as her peers to show what she is capable of in her school exams. Therefore, you may have to push for any reasonable accommodations that are open to her. Keep informed and aware of any dates and deadlines you need to know. See Chapter 3 for possible options for support in the state exams.

> 'You need to be on the ball, keeping an eye on when forms are being given in for accommodations for state exams. Plan ahead, know key dates coming up to exam years. You have to do detective work. Appeal if you think it's the wrong decision. Follow it up yourself, try to get them on the phone. That's how my son got the laptop. Apply to college for exemptions, fill in the forms, know the dates, the entitlements, the deadlines.'
>
> Yvonne's good advice

> 'Parents, fight your corner leading up to state exams – getting your waiver, a reader, a scribe – and share in the disappointment when you don't get the supports. Dates and deadlines will pass so quickly and you've missed your opportunity. Then your child is going to sit an exam where it will be really difficult for them to do as well as they should and have worked for. They won't get the marks they deserve.'
>
> Katie

And remember that a student being granted any exam accommodations, as recommended by professionals, does not mean that this student will have an unfair advantage compared to her peers. So remind others that having additional support in exams is not giving your dyslexic child an unfair advantage. They have the right to show their actual abilities and potential the same as everybody else.

## Keep things in perspective

You can be your dyslexic child's greatest asset in your role as an advocate. Be confident in that, and be encouraged by your own hard work on your child's behalf. It can be extremely stressful trying to negotiate the education system on behalf of your dyslexic child. Be prepared for times when all your efforts do not bring the outcome you were hoping for. Meetings and phone calls can be stressful, especially when there are differences of opinion on how to deal with your child's dyslexia.

Sometimes, you just have to take a step back, and accept that you cannot single-handedly transform a whole system. You cannot force teachers to understand dyslexia as you now do. However, there is no harm in suggesting the school offers specific training on dyslexia to teachers, and let them know when there is a course being organized by the Dyslexia Association or another organization. And finally, good luck!

## Takeaways from Chapter 11

- keep up with the latest developments
- communicate and negotiate on behalf of your dyslexic child
- liaise with the school at crucial points
- educate others on dyslexia
- fight for equal access to exam potential

## CHAPTER TWELVE

# Emotional Support – Fostering Self-Belief

'Those of us with dyslexia share a common thread of growing up in a society that judges us. In some cases, we have been judged as retarded in our abilities to read or do maths. In others, we are seen as less able or less intelligent. In most cases, though, the judgement is usually wrong.'[1]

Jack Horner, palaeontologist

## The Struggle for Self-Esteem

This chapter will provide various ways to help support your child's self-esteem. It looks at the difficulties faced by the dyslexic child from the early to teenage years and offers ways you can help by:

- encouraging strengths and abilities
- raising expectations
- changing the language around dyslexia
- owning it and respecting it

A definition of self-esteem: 'the extent to which we like or approve of ourselves or how worthwhile we think we are'.[2] It is bound up with 'self-concept' or 'self-belief' – how we build a picture of ourselves, which is heavily influenced by experiences at school, at home, with teachers, family and peer group.[3]

Poor self-esteem will be a significant concern for parents who are trying to support their children with dyslexia. The most, if not the only, damaging effect of dyslexia is how dyslexics perceive themselves in the world around them. This poor self-esteem is fuelled by people's ignorance of dyslexia, the constant negative language around this learning difference, and the demoralizing situations that keep reminding dyslexic children that they are not good enough and should lower their expectations.

A lack of self-esteem permeates schooling, relationships with parents and siblings, future expectations and careers. Without appropriate understanding and intervention, the negative, long-term effect on self-confidence will continue through to adult life.

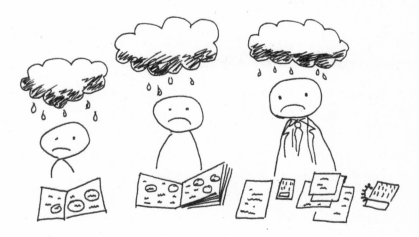

A serious aside – many studies have shown a link between poor self-esteem and juvenile crime or experimentation with drugs. A dyslexic individual who has a frustrated intelligence that is not being recognized and nurtured may find alternative routes in life. Much research has shown a high proportion of illiterate prisoners are, in fact, dyslexic, possibly as much as 30 per cent of the prison population.

People with dyslexia are not reaching their potential; their inherent abilities are not being tapped into. There is a pattern of failure that is hard to escape, and an internalized belief that the dyslexic individual is not worthy of success, not capable of facing challenges. The positive in all this is that low self-esteem or lack of self-belief is not a fixed state. Every individual with dyslexia is capable of change and taking the opportunity to raise self-confidence and belief in oneself.

## Enhancing Your Child's Self-Esteem

It is the role of a parent to combat these regular, negative experiences in school with teachers and peers, at home with siblings and in the world around the dyslexic child.

Fortunately, you can support your child's self-esteem in many significant ways, as explored in every chapter of this guide:

- knowing what dyslexia really is – Chapters 1 and 2
- practical help at home that supports academic success – Chapters 5 to 10
- being an advocate for your child – Chapters 3 and 11
- emotional support – Chapter 4

You can see that encouraging strong self-belief is a positive by-product of chapters throughout this guide; therefore, this chapter focuses on specific areas where we can grasp the opportunity to raise confidence and self-esteem.

## The Early Years

The primary school years are very exposing for the dyslexic child. There are expected milestones to reach, reading levels to get through, times tables to learn and weekly spelling tests. Challenging areas for most young pupils but, if you also have a poor short-term memory, can't do rote learning and need more time to process your thoughts, then the struggles to keep up with your peers become overwhelming, demoralizing and inevitably lead to a poor self-image.

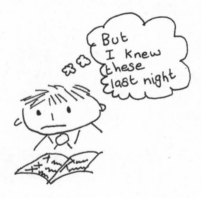

'I didn't know how to do anything until after third class. I didn't think I was good at doing anything in school.'

Caoimhe, 14, remembering her early years

'As I got older, I realized I wasn't the same level as others and that would upset me.'

Aoife, 13, remembering her early years

Dyslexic children who are assessed as 'average', 'high average' or 'superior' regarding their intelligence in an educational psychologist's report, will paradoxically consider themselves stupid and not able to succeed compared to their peers or siblings. How can this be? Surely they should be achieving equally compared with their classmates and

coming out as outstanding in certain areas of strength.
And yet a lot of primary learning sets them up to struggle and fail.

Also does a Department of Education's requirements to test children
at certain stages in their school career really reflect a dyslexic child's
intelligence and abilities? Or do these tests just reinforce a poor self-
image and an opinion that they are not capable of doing well?

## How you can help foster self-belief

### Encourage genuine strengths

Young children with dyslexia have amazing resilience when dealing
with these disappointments and frustrations every day in school. But to
build their self-confidence they must also experience competency and
success. They must feel achievement outside of these struggles.

So look at your child's strengths – what is she good at? What does she
have an innate ability to do? You now have a good insight into how people
with dyslexia have certain strengths and abilities, and you can spot these
traits in your child and help them flourish. It may be creative thinking,
good problem-solving, visual-spatial ability or language skills which
can then be used to your child's advantage in storytelling, team sports,
puzzles, making things, fixing things, playing a musical instrument,
involvement in drama, and so on.

It is crucial that you acknowledge and encourage these genuine
strengths and interests. And any successes your child experiences,
however small at times, will keep adding and adding to a stronger self-
belief.

**CASE STUDY**

**CATHAL, A PARENT OF TWO DYSLEXIC CHILDREN, GIVES HIS THOUGHTS AND ADVICE**

'In a world that will tell them that they are, at best, weird and, at worst, somehow stupid and lazy and not trying and awkward, they need to know that they are great.

'Find what they excel at and let them excel there and show the importance of that area.

'My daughter loves Art and my heart swells with pride as I see her being brilliant there, and while it doesn't make her any less dyslexic, it makes her difficulties, not less important, but less focused. My son loves Maths and wants to go on walks with me and talk about mathematical concepts.

'If your child loses their confidence it is extremely difficult to get it back. Once it has been damaged, there will always be doubt. Work hard at home to keep confidence up and fight their corner if there is ever any doubt. Allow your child to excel at what they enjoy and do not keep dragging it back to what they can't do.

'My children know more now about themselves and their abilities because of their dyslexia than many of their peers because they have had to address these questions earlier.'

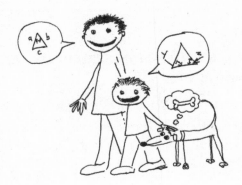

'I'm good at making things, I can draw animals – birds and dogs from my head.'

Helena, 12

'I'm good at Art, I enjoy it. I'm good at making sculptures from clay like animals and trees. I'm good at Maths. Dyslexia might hold me back with some stuff but most of them I don't want to do anyway.'

Luca, 10

'My dad would teach me secondary school Maths and I'd get it right and that would make me feel really happy. I'm a genius! I am not an idiot.'

Roan, 11

It is important that you praise and encourage your child's abilities inside and outside the academic sphere. But don't over-praise! Your child isn't stupid, she can spot over-the-top praise for something she knows isn't her best.

However, don't be overly critical when she doesn't do as well as expected. Maybe the results haven't been great but surely the effort (often four times more effort than their peers or siblings) should be recognized and given the acclaim it deserves.

<u>Raise expectations</u>

As Jack Horner, the celebrated palaeontologist, asserts at the beginning of this chapter, one of the greatest frustrations for people with dyslexia is the predominant attitude of others around them who assume dyslexics are at a terrible disadvantage and can only achieve against all odds!

You will now know, of course, that this is not the case at all. You are well aware of the inherent abilities and strengths of dyslexic individuals, and that they often succeed not despite their dyslexia but because of it.

So why lower the expectations of your dyslexic child, particularly when compared to siblings? How will that support his self-belief?

. . . . . . . . . . . . . . . . . . . . . . . . . . . . . . . . . . . . . . . . . .

If a child believes he cannot reach the expectations he may have for himself, how will he fulfil his true potential?

. . . . . . . . . . . . . . . . . . . . . . . . . . . . . . . . . . . . . . . . . .

As the number-one advocate for your child, you can educate and remind others that having dyslexia does not mean 'low ability' or 'impairment'. Your child can be challenged in his school work. If he is given the right support, he can achieve as well as and better than his peers.

. . . . . . . . . . . . . . . . . . . . . . . . . . . . . . . . . . . . . . . . . .

Never lower expectations or allow teachers or other professionals to do so.

. . . . . . . . . . . . . . . . . . . . . . . . . . . . . . . . . . . . . . . . . .

These are intelligent children who are acutely aware when they are given 'baby' work compared to the rest of the class. Yes, dyslexia has its difficulties, but with motivation, skills practice and encouragement there is no reason why dyslexic children won't succeed way above these low expectations placed on them. Keeping your child challenged in school and raising any low expectations are fundamental for a robust self-belief and a better chance of reaching potential.

Here are dyslexic children opening up about their own experiences of low expectation:

> 'I'm not expected to do well, just to pass the exam.'
>
> 'I had my hand up with a really good point, but the teacher ignored me because she didn't really expect me to come up with something amazing.'
>
> 'Friends assume I can't read or write – it really annoys me.'
>
> 'Others' attitude is really annoying . . . "How are you dyslexic? You always get higher than me." I'd really get annoyed by that and say, "Did you know Albert Einstein was dyslexic?!"'
>
> 'As a dyslexic wanting to achieve more, school can be so frustrating. You either feel you're not being seen, or you're just going into yourself because you're not achieving what you want. It can be tiring and frustrating.'

### Look at all the amazing, talented people who have dyslexia

A great boost for young dyslexics is the knowledge that other people just like them have found what they are good at and have pursued their ambitions, often because of their specific way of thinking and not despite it. Just consider some well-known dyslexics:

- Albert Einstein, Isaac Newton and Stephen Hawking, whose names are synonymous with the word 'genius'
- Charles Darwin, who transformed the way we think about the natural world
- Pablo Picasso and Andy Warhol, both extremely influential artists of the twentieth century

- Bill Gates and Steve Jobs, who have transformed modern communication for all of us
- Thomas Edison, probably the most prolific inventor of all time
- The Wright brothers and Henry Ford, who revolutionized transportation in the modern age
- Mozart and Beethoven, two of the most prolific and influential composers
- Lord Richard Rodgers, one of the most pioneering architects of the modern era
- Sportsmen and women include the cultural icon Muhammad Ali
- Entrepreneurial dyslexics include Anita Roddick, who founded The Body Shop, Tommy Hilfiger, Jo Malone, Ingvar Kamprad, who founded IKEA
- Being dyslexic is no barrier to becoming a writer, as testified by the success of Irvine Welsh, Agatha Christie, W. B. Yeats, Sir Arthur Conan Doyle, F. Scott Fitzgerald, Jules Verne, Lewis Carroll and John Irving
- And an extraordinary array of actors include Marlon Brando, Sir Anthony Hopkins, Will Smith, Keira Knightley, Orlando Bloom, Whoopi Goldberg and George Clooney

And the lists go on. The world would be a very different place without people with dyslexia.

Those often latent abilities are there to be spotted and given an opportunity to grow. You can give the space and support for your dyslexic child's confidence to flourish. It is a good idea to find out about the successful dyslexics your child admires, whether they are in the Arts, the Sciences, Sports or Business and Entrepreneurism. Make a project out of it or encourage a school project to be on a famous dyslexic. There are plenty of strong positive messages that can filter through to a dyslexic child's mind when she realizes that the people she admires are the same as her.

'It definitely helps knowing there are famous people. There are so many people I just didn't know that they're dyslexic and they're so fabulous. They've done great things. You're not stupid if you're dyslexic, you're actually pretty good.'

Roan, 11

'It boosted my confidence seeing famous people have it. I'm a big fan of Orlando Bloom. I'm glad he talks openly about his dyslexia.'

Sean, 13

'The advantage is my brain sees and puts information in my head differently, sometimes more interestingly than if I saw like everyone else.'[4]

Whoopi Goldberg, actor

'If they follow their particular dreams and what they're good at, they can be more successful at what they're good at than others. There are so many people like myself who have excelled in their individual professions who have been dyslexics.'[5]

Richard Branson, entrepreneur

'For me in my life, dyslexia has been a little bit of a blessing. It helped me find my strength and directed me towards what I really wanted to do.'[6]

Darcey Bussell, ballet dancer

## The Later School Years

Once in secondary school, and particularly if the dyslexia has gone unrecognized through the whole of primary school, low self-esteem and poor self-image can become a more complex and severe issue manifesting in a range of behaviours, such as work avoidance, aggression, playing up and withdrawal.

> 'It's a learning curve for the parents, too. We learn day by day how to deal with it and, as they grow up and change emotionally, then that changes, too – how they feel about it.'
>
> Kate, parent

A teenage dyslexic can experience a range of emotions: frustration, failure, anxiety, exhaustion, vulnerability, humiliation, demoralization and depression.

By the time a young student moves to secondary school, there could well be a pattern of thinking that is hard to change. Confidence has diminished so much there is a perceived barrier to learning and an inability to focus on strengths or positive feedback. Repeated failures, however minor, at home and at school can devastate self-esteem.

A strong self-concept in these teenage years is hard to achieve for anyone, and as schoolwork becomes more demanding the message often received is that they are just not able. They can't help focusing on the moments that prove in their own eyes their uselessness.

Frustratingly, it is true that a dyslexic student experiences a lot of failure. Processing and learning new material is a challenge, along with failing to read or spell at the expected level. They are in a daily cycle of failure and can be so low in self-worth that they give up completely. If they are not achieving, then why bother? Their attitude becomes highly negative as a result – they might as well attempt less and then they will fail less. They become less willing to try a new task for fear of failure. What's the point in trying?

---

**CASE STUDY**

**TADHG, AGED 15, REFLECTS ON HIS OWN BEHAVIOUR
AND FEELINGS**

'It's great to realize that I'm not slow but it still hasn't really sunk in that I'm not slow. It will never really sink in. I know I'm smart, I have a high IQ but that doesn't matter in school.

'All those experiences in primary school – still there, still the feelings are going to be there for ever – no one will ever notice that I'm struggling with something. I try to hide things by not caring. I became a troublemaker. Instead of trying, I'd give them as little as possible. I'd rather be classed as lazy than be classed as stupid. I'd always underachieve. I'd rather not do it than fail.

'We will hide it if we get it wrong – if I got it wrong, I'd crumple it up and say I didn't do it. It was easier to get into trouble than look stupid in front of someone. That's why I'd always clash with teachers. I got 62 notes home saying I hadn't done it.'

---

## Supporting a Dyslexic Teenager at Home

Three factors are critical when supporting your dyslexic teenager: (i) encourage genuine strengths; (ii) praise effort; and (iii) raise expectations.

Just as there are many opportunities for humiliation and failure in school, sadly there can equally be these experiences at home. Without realizing it, parents and other members of the household can reinforce this poor self-concept.

....................................

Praise and encourage effort rather than focusing on the negatives, the bad results and the weaknesses.

....................................

Home should be a refuge from those negative school experiences. However, the well-intentioned parent may become a 'teacher' at home adding to those feelings of inadequacy from outside. The best-intentioned parents can inadvertently fuel the stresses and feelings of incompetence as they become exasperated by their dyslexic child's forgetfulness and perceived inability to study. Your dyslexic child's home environment needs to be calm and supportive, encouraging genuine abilities and interests.

....................................

It is crucial that talents are recognized and developed.

....................................

Yes, the academic struggles must be looked after, but with the support of home there are many possible areas of interest where your dyslexic child can experience confidence and success. When strengths are recognized and shared confidently then the difficulties in school will be accepted with more resilience.

> 'Although she has dyslexia, I can now see that it is really just one part of her and doesn't hold her back at all. She actually did a brilliant junior certificate and was so amazed by her results that she had to keep checking that her name was on the top of the page, as in she thought perhaps she was looking at someone else's results! It was touching and sad, and happy all at the same time for me. She is very creative, hugely into singing, dancing, musical theatre and wants to be involved in that as a career. She is hugely dedicated.'
>
> Niamh, parent of a dyslexic daughter

'They can absolutely do everything. It hasn't made a huge difference. All the boys are logical thinkers, talented in music, business, engineering, cooking. You look at subject choices very closely. You just focus on the strong subjects all the time.'

Yvonne, parent of three dyslexic sons

'You can dart between the raindrops to get where you want to go, and it will not hold you back.'[7]

Steven Spielberg

## How can you deal with comparisons with non-dyslexic siblings?

This is often an area of concern for dyslexic individuals who have younger or older siblings. However much parents may tell their dyslexic child how able she is, the dyslexic child will still be sensitive to comparisons with a sibling who has no 'problem' with learning and study, and may be perceived as 'the intelligent one'.

To add salt to the wounds, the young dyslexic may also have teachers who compare her lack of achievement to her sibling who does well in tests and rote learning. So do try not to compare your dyslexic child to your other children, in terms of when milestones are reached or any perceived educational difficulties.

'I can't stress enough that you can't compare them to your other children – they will take it to heart. You can't tell them they're worse than someone else because they'll believe it instantly. They already think they are worse than everyone. Even if they don't show it they do think that, because they're dyslexic, so never compare them to other people, just don't do it. If parents are saying it, then what are other people saying, who aren't related to you, who don't care about your feelings? What are they saying behind your back?'

Tadhg, on the sibling issue

These comparisons can be acutely felt by your dyslexic son or daughter. It is very easy to internalize how we feel we are perceived by significant people in our lives.

You could also overcompensate with your dyslexic child, and this has its own pitfalls. Overprotection of your dyslexic child can disempower him and weaken his self-concept, causing anxiety.

> 'Don't pamper! It reinforces the idea in the child's head that they're less intelligent than their brother or sister. Encourage what they're good at and deflect from what siblings are good at.'
>
> Advice from Mike, with non-dyslexic siblings

Look at the sibling issue from an alternative viewpoint – have you considered that your non-dyslexic children could be jealous of the extra attention you are giving your dyslexic child? Your dyslexic child, in their eyes, is being lavished with extra help outside school and lots of one-to-one time with you practising paired reading, helping with homework and so on.

> 'There is the other side – my brother hated me because I got more attention from Mum. My mum spent extra time with me reading. So there can be certain jealousy from siblings having a dyslexic sister or brother. They just need some extra help, not that parents love them more!'
>
> Mike

It is a fine line, and the sibling issue is one where it is impossible to have one answer. You will know your children and what works for them. The best you can do is to be aware of how having a dyslexic child can affect sibling relationships. Of course, you could be in a household full of dyslexics, so that makes life easier!

## Owning and Respecting Dyslexia

Even when a dyslexic student is succeeding in her chosen subjects and on her way to achieving her goals, her self-esteem can still be fragile. She will not believe the assurances of others, particularly parents. It is important to respect your child's dyslexia; it is part of who she is and how she sees the world. Encourage 'owning it'!

When you accept the strengths and advantages of your child's dyslexia, then you automatically accept a huge part of who she is, and that is important for healthy self-esteem.

### Talk openly about dyslexia

It is extremely important that your child talks about her dyslexia to others, freely, without embarrassment, and you must follow suit. Giving your child the space to explain her way of seeing the world will be an enlightening experience for you, too. Take your child's lead.

This is giving the strong message that dyslexia is nothing to be ashamed of; in fact, it can be celebrated and your child can educate others with that message. The last thing your child needs is any whiff of shame or disappointment emanating from you. You have got to change your perceptions of dyslexia, change your language around it, educate others and be strong in your conviction for your child's sake.

> 'You can still do everything you want to do. You will have strengths. Don't let it get you down. If you think it's going to affect your life, you're wrong. Tell someone if you're dyslexic. It's not going to affect how your friends think of you.'
>
> Dylan's advice, 16

## Change the language around dyslexia

As emphasized right from the beginning of this guide, any notion of a disability and the language usually associated with such a label has to be ruled out. We must change the language around dyslexia so we can really fully support a child with this 'learning difference'. We need to dispel that negative language – 'despite <u>suffering</u> from dyslexia they finally <u>overcame their disability</u>.' Although it is great to hear about famous dyslexics via the media, it is infuriating for the dyslexic individual to observe these celebratory stories couched in negative language and hear how the successful dyslexic succeeded '<u>despite this terrible affliction</u>' and '<u>against all odds</u>!'

Well-meaning comments such as '<u>it must be a terrible struggle</u>' also do not help matters. With such debilitating language around this learning difference, it is no wonder that dyslexics have to put up with sympathy and worse – patronizing pity. How frustrating for an intelligent and ambitious individual.

They don't want pity or sympathy, they want to be respected and celebrated for their different way of processing and seeing the world. It is part of who they are and how they think.

And you need to be on board with that, to then educate others in changing the language from 'disability' to a <u>different ability</u>, a <u>learning difference</u> rather than 'difficulty'. By transforming the dominant notions of dyslexia, we can boost the confidence of the dyslexic child, raise expectations and nurture self-belief.

You can help facilitate your dyslexic child to see the benefits of these different ways of thinking and processing the world around him.

Understanding, accepting and actually celebrating these differences will help your dyslexic child to see his dyslexia in a positive light. It may well be that it is you who needs more convincing than your talented dyslexic child. Either way, give him space and encouragement to 'own' his dyslexia; after all, it belongs to him, it is part of how he sees the world.

Look at the huge number of people with dyslexia who have been the innovators in their chosen field and have proven themselves to be at the top of their game, from Leonardo da Vinci to Picasso, from Mozart to John Lennon, from Isaac Newton to Stephen Hawking, from Walt Disney to Steven Spielberg.

> **'Don't ever let people put you down for being dyslexic. Being dyslexic is actually an advantage, and has helped me greatly in life.'[8]**
>
> Richard Branson in a letter to a 9-year-old girl with dyslexia

Here are young people celebrating their dyslexia:

> 'I openly speak about dyslexia, I connect more with people.'
>
> Sean, 13

> 'I can think a bit differently to other people. Sometimes everyone has the same ideas but you may have a more abstract view. You can come up with a different idea.'
>
> Molly, 18

> 'I feel being dyslexic has made me understand people more. It may sound silly, but I'll never judge someone if they don't get something straight away. And I help people who struggle because I know what it is like. It's made me a creative thinker. It's made me more ambitious

to do well and prove people, who have the wrong idea of dyslexia, wrong, too.'

Emma, 16

'I think I'm a confident person because of my dyslexia. When I wasn't doing well at spelling and reading, I was excelling at keeping up with the class in other aspects. I was really intelligent when it came to certain things and it showed to me that I am so capable. I do think dyslexia has given me skills that have benefited me in every aspect. I like my dyslexia.'

Katie, 19

## Takeaways from Chapter 12

- encourage genuine interests and strengths
- don't allow any lowering of expectations
- recognize and praise effort
- encourage your dyslexic child to own it
- transform the language around dyslexia

# A FINAL WORD – DYSLEXIA BEYOND THE SCHOOL YEARS

## After the School Years

School can be a tough time for dyslexic children, and this can be due to various reasons – a lack of understanding of dyslexia, a lack of resources or intervention and appropriate support. Parents can only do their best when they are up against entrenched attitudes to this learning difference and conflicting ideas on what is best for their child.

Be comforted by the fact that you are making a difference for your dyslexic child with your support. And after sometimes gruelling years in school, there are ever-increasing opportunities for assistive technology and ways to pursue genuine strengths and abilities.

Once secondary school has been completed, a dyslexic young person is free to pursue interests and possible college courses. You will have done your bit by encouraging interests and abilities outside of school, making sure no low expectations are placed upon your dyslexic teenager and by helping to change attitudes towards dyslexia.

'Encouraging self-developed interests is important. Having interests which go beyond the scope of school, these are the things which have made my life have comfort and passion. The things when I was struggling that I could turn to. Video games, reading, art and walking have all been the way I see myself. If I only worked at school and did mediocre at leaving cert (the Leaving Certificate examinations), then that would be the only value of myself.

'But I valued myself by the fact I'd started writing a comic book during 6th Year and was far more proud of this. I only did an OK leaving cert but, at the end of the day, it was enough to get me into college and figure out where I wanted to go from there. It didn't serve to reflect my worth because I didn't allow it.'

Ben, graduate

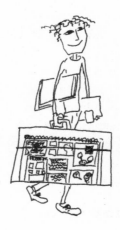

You now know that dyslexia is not a terrible 'ordeal' to be 'endured' or 'overcome'. Yes, dyslexia has its challenges but, with the right intervention and support, unexpected advantages and qualities can be harnessed and encouraged, particularly in the post-school years. Your encouragement and support will have been invaluable.

'I feel like an advantage I have over other people is being able to see things from an alternative perspective. Your 'edge' is abstract thinking, determination, a slightly different perspective on things. I studied Philosophy in college. I've always found it really easy to think in the abstract and, at school, you never get to think in the abstract, so sometimes I felt stupid at school but not at college. I could have

proper conversations and it didn't matter I didn't know what
8 x 6 is.'

Niamh, graduate

'There wasn't anything to get through; it isn't a 'diagnosis'. It's not something that will really affect you the rest of your life. I focused on the things I was really good at and that I really enjoyed. I'm fairly ambitious, I have loads of ideas.'

Katie, graduate

'I've never felt that I couldn't go to college and do anything I want, because I've had supportive parents. The main thing the child knows is that they have the support to reach their goals regardless of being dyslexic. It is important for a child to know that the parent is actually there and they will do anything they possibly can to help them. Parents are the best asset a child can have in those first few critical years – if active and committed to the child's welfare, the child can do literally anything they want.'

Mike, graduate

## Changing Attitudes to Dyslexia

'Word blindness' was a term coined in the nineteenth century and still heard today as a way to explain dyslexia. Dyslexic children are still being labelled as 'slow', 'lazy', 'unteachable' or 'remedial'. These misunderstandings about dyslexia will continue, so be prepared to come up against outdated attitudes, such as: 'It's just a reading and spelling difficulty' ... 'It doesn't really exist' ... 'It's just an excuse for laziness' ... 'It's a middle-class disease'.

There have been positive changes in attitude towards dyslexia recently, supported by scientific research and famous people talking about their dyslexia in the media. But there is still a way to go. Your role is to educate others, change the language around dyslexia and help establish a view of dyslexia for the twenty-first century.

'It depends on the person, when I say I'm dyslexic.  People say, "Oh, you can't read properly and you can't write properly." That's what they think, and I say, "No! Sometimes it takes longer to learn stuff but some things you remember really well." "What did you have for dinner?" And I'd have no idea what I had for dinner!'

Juliette, 17

'I'm not ashamed to be dyslexic, but people in the past would have been. I talk to my friends about it. Some people still think you are stupid but it's not their fault, they just never had the opportunity to learn about it.'

Tadhg, 15

'My teacher will never believe the brightest person in the class could be dyslexic. Other people are open to it. When I am older, my generation will get it. They will know they can be better at some subjects.'

Sarah, 15

There are two ways to look at dyslexia – you can see it as a learning disability characterized by its difficulties and its 'impediments'; or you can see it as a learning difference – a different way of processing and seeing the world. We can then open up to the opportunities and strengths and not just accept the assumed struggles and barriers.

Being dyslexic gives you remarkable advantages, in that your brain works in a different way. We need to emphasize the abilities and unique opportunities that dyslexia can give. And these are not platitudes – there is enough scientific research, observations and the experiences of so many talented and successful dyslexics that confirm this advantage.

We can begin by changing the language. Let's reframe dyslexia and transform peoples' perceptions – a 'rebranding' to highlight it as a difference to be celebrated and nurtured for all our good.

There are positive transformations happening, but there is still plenty of work to be done to change the predominant negative view of people with dyslexia. What would our world be without the talents and vision of these exceptional minds?

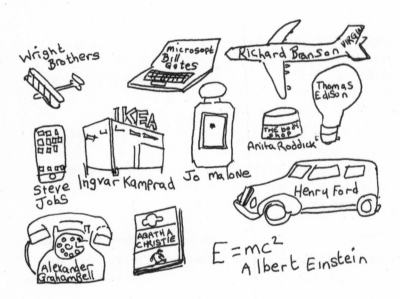

'The world without dyslexia would be old, depressing and boring. We wouldn't have IKEA!'

Roan, 11

'I know I can talk to everyone now and I won't be judged.'

Aoife, 13

'I see the future for dyslexia a lot better than it used to be . . . the future will keep on getting better I think.'

Luca, 10

## Possible Co-Existing Difficulties

### Dyspraxia, or Developmental Co-ordination Disorder (DCD)

A neurological issue affecting fine and/or gross motor co-ordination, making it hard to plan and co-ordinate movement.

<u>Signs and symptoms of dyspraxia</u>

- gross motor issues with balance and co-ordination
- fine motor issues with handwriting, an awkward pencil grip
- organization and time-management difficulties
- easily distracted and fidgety
- difficulty with planning and focusing

### Dysgraphia

An issue with the ability to write, often making handwriting messy and illegible. It can be a difficulty with fine motor skills and remembering sequences when writing.

<u>Signs and symptoms of dysgraphia</u>

- fine motor issues, an awkward pencil grip
- slow and laboured writing
- inconsistent letter shape and size, and poor spacing
- often illegible writing, particularly when tired or rushed

- experiencing pain in the wrist and up the arm, even after a relatively short piece of writing such as a short paragraph

Occupational therapy and other tools and strategies, such as those for a child with dyslexia, can make a difference for children with dyspraxia and dysgraphia. Assistive technology and everyday use of a laptop or similar will be the best solution for most concerns.

## Irlen Syndrome or Scotopic Sensitivity

A visual perception problem affecting the reading of text and aggravated by environmental stressors such as fluorescent light. An individual with Irlen Syndrome has an unusual sensitivity to specific frequencies and wavelengths of the white light spectrum. It is undetected by standard eye tests.

<u>Signs and symptoms of Irlen Syndrome or Scotopic Sensitivity</u>
- bothered by the glare of a white page, computer screens, fluorescent lights
- difficulty reading as the print appears to blur, move, swirl, flash, disappear
- feeling tension and fatigue when reading
- physical reactions include sore eyes, watery eyes, frequent headaches, migraines, stomach ache
- difficulty focusing and retaining content of a reading passage

The discomfort can be reduced with the use of specific coloured transparencies, or 'overlays', over the written text. Tinted filters worn as glasses or contact lenses can calm the physical environment and aid memory and concentration. A specialist in this area will help to prescribe the specific filter needed. (See www.irlen.com for more information.)

# ENDNOTES

## Preliminary pages

1 Orlando Bloom, interview with Dr Harold Koplewicz for the Child Mind Institute, 2010. Reproduced with permission of the CMI

## Chapter 1

1 Report of the Task Force on Dyslexia, The Dyslexia Association of Ireland, 2001

2 J. R. Horner, 'The Extraordinary Characteristics of Dyslexia', originally published in <u>Perspectives on Language and Literacy</u>, © International Dyslexia Association, Inc, July 2008

3 Benjamin Zephaniah, <u>Creative, Successful, Dyslexic: 23 High Achievers Share their Stories</u>, ed. Margaret Rooke, Jessica Kingsley Publishers, 2016. Reproduced with permission of Jessica Kingsley Publishers Ltd through PLSclear

## Chapter 2

1 Eddie Izzard, <u>Creative, Successful, Dyslexic: 23 High Achievers Share their Stories</u>, ed. Margaret Rooke, Jessica Kingsley Publishers, 2016. Reproduced with permission of Jessica Kingsley Publishers Ltd through PLSclear

## Chapter 4

1 Benjamin Zephaniah, <u>Creative, Successful, Dyslexic: 23 High Achievers Share their Stories</u>, ed. Margaret Rooke, Jessica Kingsley

Publishers, 2016. Reproduced with permission of Jessica Kingsley Publishers Ltd through PLSclear

2    Steven Spielberg, interview with Quinn Bradlee for the Friends of Quinn website, www.friendsofquinn.com, a project of the National Center for Learning Disabilities, New York

## Chapter 7

1    Agatha Christie, An Autobiography, Collins. 1977. Reproduced with permission of Agatha Christie Ltd

2    Excerpts from Roald Dahl's school reports, the Roald Dahl archive at the Roald Dahl Museum and Story Centre. Reproduced with permission of the Roald Dahl Literary Estate

## Chapter 12

1    J. R. Horner, 'The Extraordinary Characteristics of Dyslexia', originally published in Perspectives on Language and Literacy, © the International Dyslexia Association, Inc., July 2008

2    Gross, R. & McIlveen, R. Psychology: A New Introduction. London, Hodder & Stoughton, 1998

3    Mortimer, T. Dyslexia and Learning Style: A Practitioner's Handbook, Whurr Publishers, 2003

4    Whoopi Goldberg, interview with Quinn Bradlee for the Friends of Quinn website, www.friendsofquinn.com, a project of the National Center for Learning Disabilities, New York

5    Richard Branson, reproduced with permission of Virgin.com

6    Darcey Bussell, Creative, Successful, Dyslexic: 23 High Achievers Share their Stories, ed. Margaret Rooke, Jessica Kingsley Publishers, 2016. Reproduced with permission of Jessica Kingsley Publishers Ltd through PLSclear

7    Steven Spielberg, interview with Quinn Bradlee for the Friends of Quinn website, www.friendsofquinn.com, a project of the National Center for Learning Disabilities, New York

8    Richard Branson, reproduced with permission of Virgin.com

## ACKNOWLEDGEMENTS

My grateful thanks to all the students and parents who shared their stories and advice for this book, and to my students, past and present, whose insights, determination, creativity and humour continue to inspire.

I wish to thank Nikki Read and all at Little, Brown Book Group, and the Society of Authors. I would also like to thank the illustrator Danielle Sheehy and express gratitude to Kieran O'Connor Design for all their help.

A special thank you to Anthony Robinson for all his input and encouragement from the beginning.

# INDEX